A Word from Paul

If I were to summarize the secret to excellent health—the rrari. A Ferrari is the archetype ance machines ever made. It is body as you would a Ferrari—using only the best fuel and regularly taking it to the best mechanic for maintenance—your body will give you ten times what you put into it, for the duration of your life. So ask yourself, "Do I treat my body like a Ferrari or a Pinto?"

Your body is a high performance sports car transporting you through life. It is the vehicle you use to experience everything. If your vehicle is in excellent condition, your life experiences will be more full and complete. If you choose to take average care of your high performance sports car, you should only expect an average life experience. The more you respect your body and care for it the more magic you will experience.

Lean Health tells the story of how I went from having average health to having exceptional health. I achieved this exceptional health in just one year. These are the four things that define exceptional health for me:

1. Most of my life I was over 210 pounds. Now I find it easy to maintain 165, which is the correct weight for my height of 5'10". *(Go to the link at the end of this section to watch Excellent Health has Many Benefits video)*

2. When I go to the doctor for a checkup, he says, "You look amazing and your health is excellent. What are you doing?"

3. I have a strong, muscular body with a chiseled abdomen; something that was just a dream before.

4. Finally and most important, it is easy to sustain exceptional health. After a full year of living healthy, I have no temptation to backslide into any unhealthy habits. I just have a total love affair with serving and taking care of my greatest customer…my body! *(Go to the link at the end of this section to watch my One Year Lean video)*

2secondlean.com/lh-word

Foreword
by Jeffrey K. Liker

When Jim Womack was working on "The Machine that Changed the World" he was struggling to name this remarkable phenomenon that Toyota seemed to exemplify.

Toyota was thinking long-term; innovating, designing and building high quality cars at a steady pace, with very little inventory or other waste, while claiming their purpose was to contribute to society. It sounded too good to be true! A graduate student at the time, John Krafcik, suggested he call this unusual way of thinking and behaving "lean" because Toyota was doing more of everything with less of everything, like a lean athlete.

Now we come full circle and Paul has provided wondrous imagery of what it is like to live a lean lifestyle. And he is able to provide himself as an example. He is on his lean journey at work and is now extending that to a lean personal lifestyle.

This is also a lean book—written crisply, clearly and in a way that engages us from the first line. I love the Ferrari metaphor. Take care of your body like you would take care of your very expensive and beautiful red Ferrari. It raises the irony that we may value things more than we do our own bodies.

Toyota today presents their own way as having two pillars—respect for people and continuous improvement. Paul's book brings to mind respect for ourselves, including the impact we have on the world and continuously improving ourselves.

Continuous improvement means exactly what it says—never stop or pause. A lean lifestyle suggests that we do not take vacations from living healthy and do not proceed in fits and starts. Most diet fads lead to unusual eating patterns to lose a lot of weight, and then fight a losing battle to maintain the lower weight. In "The Toyota Way" when I talk about leveling the workload I use the analogy of the tortoise and the hare. A lean lifestyle is more like the tortoise—slow, steady and consistent. This is automatically self-sustaining.

I had a similar experience to what Paul describes, though at a much lower level. When I reached my mid-50s a friend suggested I try her personal trainer. I had been creeping up in weight every year and saw a photo of myself in a tee shirt and it frightened me to see my belly hanging out over my belt. I went to the gym and began working with the personal trainer—a petite woman who was much more gentle on me then Paul's trainer. I explained my weight loss goal and she made it simple. Only two things matter in weight loss—calories you take in minus calories you burn.

Over time she gave me eating tips. For the last six years I have maintained daily workouts, personal training for 1 hour 2-3 times a week, walking an 18 hole golf course every chance I get and eating more healthy then I used to. I get a fair share of compliments on how I look. But I use artificial sweetener, my workouts are still on the treadmill, I do not measure anything and I take over-the-counter drugs. I do not have a six-pack and have not climbed to Mount Everest Base Camp.

As you read Paul's description of how he is leading a lean lifestyle, think of it as a source of inspiration like Toyota is to many organizations throughout the world. Toyota thinks of the Toyota Way as true North, something they never can live up to 100%, but as providing a direction they aspire to. Paul is giving us a powerful true North direction. Anyone who does half of what Paul is describing will find themselves happier and healthier, at least that is what I am telling myself.

As I was writing this, my wife sent me an email with an appropriate quote that happens to be from one of the leading advocates of holistic medicine:

"Every time you are tempted to react in the same old way, ask if you want to be a prisoner of the past or a pioneer of the future." ~Deepak Chopra

Paul is providing a sensible vision of a desirable future for us all. It has already inspired me to make some changes in my own life: more pushups as part of my daily exercise, more vegetables and fruit. I am right now at an airport and after reading the book selected a chef salad instead of a barbeque sandwich.

So please read this book, reflect and enjoy. What do you want your life to look like down the road? What one positive step can you take to start on a new path? Paul suggests it gets easier and at some point exercise and healthy eating are joyous experiences.

    Jeffrey K. Liker
    Author of The Toyota Way

2secondlean.com/lh-foreword

Word on the Street

After my 18th birthday, a restaurant owner at the time, I started gaining weight. I gained 4 pounds per year to be precise. Fast forward 30 years and the math becomes obvious. Obese was an understatement at a weight of 310 pounds. Then comes this 2 Second Lean Health process outlined by Paul's trials and tribulations. It took a little while to "get it" but when I did, the **rockets started firing**. I have managed to lose 4 pounds a week over the past 10 weeks! Are you kidding me? I would never, in a million years, have thought this was possible. When I am done, I will be back at my high school weight and will have added 20 active years to my life. What a gift! This is a must-do-type book. After you break through the barriers that Paul describes, you will never look at your life the same way. Paul may be a Ferrari, but I am the Space Shuttle Discovery!

George Trachilis, P.Eng., Author of OEM Principles of Lean Thinking, President & CEO, Lean Leadership Institute

In his new book, "Lean Health," Paul Akers presents a relentlessly logical, "elegant" approach to improving one's own personal state of health. **It's CLEAR.** His book is loaded with specific examples. A favorite of mine is "the picture diet." **It's ATTAINABLE.** Everything he suggests is possible for all of us. Paul does a great job of challenging the excuses we make when we try to convince ourselves that in some circumstances—travel, for example—healthy practices aren't possible. He proves they are. **It PAYS OFF more than it COSTS.** By making this approach simple and fun, Paul takes the "cost" out of the recipe. By sharing the benefits of his own journey, from being in the best shape of his life down to the exquisite tastes of non-processed, natural foods, fruits and vegetables, we can taste the payoff for making healthy changes in our own daily practices. Simply by reading this book, I have bought into launching my own Lean Health journey. Once you read it, so will you.

Doug Walker, Author of A-Ha! Performance: Building and Managing a Self-Motivate Workforce, 2007, Wiley Press

I love and respect Paul and I know his sincerity. He has not written this book to make money. He has written this book because the Lean Health process has worked so well for him and he knows it will work the same way for you. Over the last number of years, Paul has become a master of Lean. **His company, FastCap, is probably the best Lean company in America.** He produces products with very high quality, at very low cost and with very fast delivery. It is the model of "Just in Time." It follows the principles established by the Toyota Corporation. Every person at FastCap is a leader. Every person there creates an improvement idea every single day. The company is very well-organized; everything has an exact place; the floors are spotless; even the bathroom is the cleanest I have ever seen in America. Paul has made a showcase of his company and now he has made his physical body a showcase for you to follow. Now, keep it simple. In fact, Paul's major message in life is to keep it simple. His advice in the book is not complicated—no, not at all. Just look at the book as a cookbook. It is a cookbook to create a new you.

**Norman Bodek, Author of The Harada Method,
83 years old and as spry as ever**

Over the last several years I have invested considerable time in my mental, spiritual and physical health. I exercise almost every day and as a vegetarian I thought I ate fairly well. But as I crossed into my 50's, the extra weight still crept on. When Paul shared his physical transformation and the method he used, his concept of **"your body is the customer"** aligned with the customer-centric thinking I've embraced for decades as a Lean manufacturing proponent. Paul's pointers are easy to understand, easy to implement and, perhaps most importantly, easy to sustain. I quickly realized I was underestimating portion sizes and distorting the nutrition/exercise balance. By embracing Paul's Lean Health concepts - and, quite honestly, lifestyle - the positive changes have come quickly. I am adding value to my body, my customer.

Kevin Meyer, Co-Founder and Partner of Gemba Academy LLC.

If you find keeping a diet hard, this book is for you. With the plethora of dieting books in the world it's hard to imagine how anyone could carve out a niche. But that is what Paul Akers has done! He did what is missing in every other dieting book. The how. **How to get the motivation** to keep to one. Anyone eager to keep a diet who is not eager to keep a diet will find the solution to why every previous diet failed them in Paul's magnificent book. Paul not only lays out a clear recipe for healthy eating, but brilliantly explains the method to create the motivation to keep to it. Other than preparing the food for you, Paul lays it all out for us - thank you!

Rabbi Stephen Baars, Author, Executive Director of Aish Seminars

2secondlean.com/lh-street

Lean™
Health
Aging in Reverse

Paul A. Akers

FastCap Press

Copyright © 2015 by FastCap Press
All rights reserved,
including the right of reproduction
in whole or in part in any form.

For information about special discounts for bulk purchases, please contact
Paul Akers: 888-443-3748 or paul@goleanhealth.com

Written by Paul Akers
First printing, December 2015
Manufactured in the United States of America

2 Second Lean Health comes in ALL flavors

You can read it or get even more insight by watching the videos on the YouTube channel Lean Health. Or listen to the expanded Audio-Book with extra "off-script" inspiration and added stories of innovation.

**Check out 2secondlean.com for all
the latest Lean Ideas**

2secondlean.com/lh

Acknowledgments

Editors

Will Hutchens, Leanne Akers and Lori Turley who edited the original manuscript.

Graphics & Book Layout

Jayme Newby

Special Thanks

To all my Lean Health thinking friends all over the world that contributed so much to make this book everything it is. Jeffrey Liker, Ashley Bailey, Joe Rogers, George Trachilis, Greg Glebe, Dana May, Doug Walker Rabbi Stephen Baars, Alex Gaertner, Glenn Bostock, Scott Berry, Michael Althoff, Nick Kocelj, Doug Scoggins, Mark and Sherri Rosenberger, Norman Bodek, Karl Wadensten, Filipe Marques, Ty Lane, Mike Wroblewski, Metin Palik, Kelly Barlow and John Anderson

Special, Special Thanks

Paloma Cury, for giving me the ultimatum for writing the book and not letting me weasel out of it. Her direct approach and winsome smile is irresistible.

Contents

Preface
Chapter 1:   A Perfect Night in Germany   13
Chapter 2:   The Answer   16
Chapter 3:   Everest Base Camp   25
Chapter 4:   The Results   31
Chapter 5:   How Could I Be So Stupid?   34
Chapter 6:   We are All Addicts   38
Chapter 7:   Never Sick   44
Chapter 8:   The Four Things I Learned from Doug   47
Chapter 9:   Convoluted Chemistry   51
Chapter 10: Traveling is Easy   53
Chapter 11: The Big Deception   56
Chapter 12: The Picture Diet   59
Chapter 13: Lean PD App   62
Chapter 14: To Log or Not to Log?   65
Chapter 15: Racing in the Rain   68
Chapter 16: The Voice of Others   73
Chapter 17: Roadblocks   79
Chapter 18: Lead or Follow   84
Chapter 19: Discipline or Intelligence   88
Chapter 20: Building a Lean Team   92
             A Typical Day for Paul
             Twenty-One Stages of Lean Health
             Questions & Answers

2secondlean.com/lh-contents

What's This?

This green bar is a link that will take you to all the awesome videos Paul has created on his Lean Health journey. Each chapter has loads of insight and inspiring stories that will get you all excited to try this new Lean Health lifestyle.

2secondlean.com

Step 1
Type the web-link into your browser.

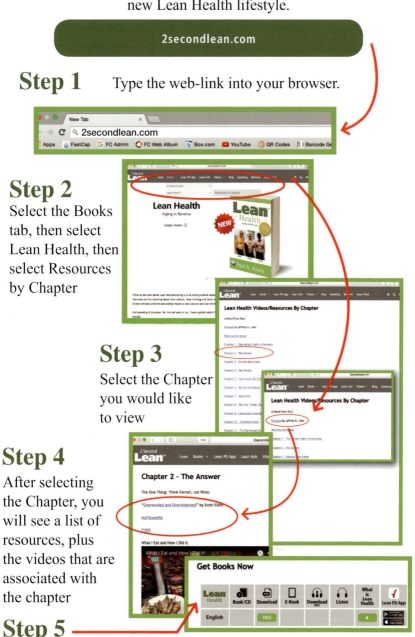

Step 2
Select the Books tab, then select Lean Health, then select Resources by Chapter

Step 3
Select the Chapter you would like to view

Step 4
After selecting the Chapter, you will see a list of resources, plus the videos that are associated with the chapter

Step 5
Under the downloads tab you can find all available versions of Lean Health **FOR FREE**

— Preface —
Who is your Customer?

As a business owner and entrepreneur, one of the most important ideas I have learned is the importance of loving your customer. My company provides services and products to our customers, and without them, *I am out of business*. However, in order for my business to be relevant, first the customer has to *want* what I have to offer. Once I understood how important customers were to my business, I came to appreciate and cherish them. I learned to love them and they reciprocated. When I say love, I mean to cherish, respect and improve everything for their benefit.

In the Lean world, we live and breathe to deliver a continuous stream of quality and value to our customers. The customer is not a part of our business, the customer *IS* our business. We are obsessed with continuous improvement and the elimination of waste. We do this so we can increase quality and let value flow to the customer assuring that we maintain a long term, mutually prosperous relationship; characterized by a deep and reverent respect.

As I wrote this book, I asked myself the question, "Who is the customer in the Lean Health scenario?" It was easy for me to identify the customer because all I did was ask, "Who is getting the short end of the stick? Who's calling the shots?" It became so clear to me that I was the business owner that was screwing my customer...my body! Wow...when I put this together I realized that I needed to make sure I reestablished proper and respectful love of my newly discovered customer. My body is my #1 customer!

As I began to understand the relationship between me and my newly discovered customer, everything changed. The moment this concept connected with total clarity deep inside of me, the quality of my life accelerated at a more rapid rate than I could have ever imagined.

All of a sudden, I considered how everything I put in my mouth would affect my customer, just like the fuel I put in my Ferrari would affect its performance. I started asking, "Is this good for my customer? What have I done to support my customer today?" I stopped being mindless and I became mindful of my cherished customer (my body)!

In the business relationship, if you treat a customer poorly they are apt to find someone else sooner or later. In the Lean Health relationship, the customer (your body) is stuck with you. If you can continue to abuse your loyal customer, they will take it as long as they can, sooner or later they will just give up. If you choose to make an intelligent decision to nurture and care for your customer, it will reward you with a positive mind-set, confidence, more energy than you could have ever dreamed possible, a boundless mental attitude, superior physical health, a longer life span, countless admirers that marvel at how someone your age could look so good. Is it worth the effort? The irony is the small amount of effort to achieve exceptional health is significantly less than dealing with all the travails of poor or average health. At the end of the day, understanding that my body is the most important customer has been a true awakening.

So welcome to Lean Health. As you read this book, use the filter that every decision you make about the food you eat and the degree to which you move, affects the most important customer in your life...your body!

Chapter 1

A Perfect Night in Germany

At eight o'clock on a pleasant August evening, I was sitting at an outdoor café in Baden-Baden, Germany, one of the most beautiful places in the world. Across from me sat two of the most amazing people I've ever met, Alex and Paloma, from Mercedes-Benz in Germany. We had just spent the last three days together, touring the Stuttgart Mercedes plant and test driving a spectacular S-Class Mercedes around Germany and France. We were bringing our journey to an end in this beautiful little city of Baden-Baden, where we sat chatting over a fantastic meal, recalling the high points of our recent adventure.

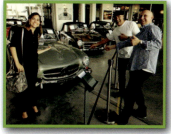

Paloma, Alex and I in Germany

As I savored my fresh tomatoes, mozzarella and parmesan-sprinkled broccoli, Paloma looked over at me and said, "Paul, when are you going to write your next book?"

"I would really love to, but I'm so busy," I replied.

I asked, "Why, Paloma, why should I write the book?" She replied, "I was waiting for my healthy food and realized you helped us change our way of thinking so fast, just three days of being with you. I thought you needed to pass on your thinking to everyone, so you should write a book.

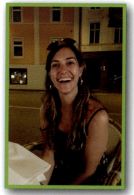

Paloma, 2 minutes after she asked me "Paul when are you going to write your next book?"

"Come on," Paloma said, her beautiful Brazilian accent coaxing me along. "You need to do it. You need to start now and write one chapter a night."

I looked at her in disbelief, "I am in the middle of a two-month trip around the world, teaching and

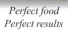

Perfect food Perfect results

training people in eight countries on how to implement Lean. I'm capturing everything I do on video, because before I left, Mel Damski, a well-known movie producer, asked me to document the entire trip for a new television program called *Lean around the World*. I also have to manage my company FastCap (a Lean manufacturing business back home in Washington State). I'm completely swamped and you're telling me you want me to also write a book? Are you crazy?"

"You'll find a way," she replied, much more confident than me.

It's hard to believe that a single person could be so influential in another person's life. I really did not want to add anything else to my plate; however, less than a minute later, a voice inside me said, "Hey Paul, practice what you preach. Go out and change the world."

So I gave in. After all, it wouldn't hurt to at least type out an outline. I pulled out my phone, and over the next 4-5 minutes typed out the titles of twelve chapters explaining my health journey. I felt empowered by typing out those chapter headings in such a short time.

"What do you think it should be called?" I asked her. "Healthy Lean? Lean Health?

I think 'Lean Health' sounds good," she replied. *(Go to the link at the end of this chapter to watch Paloma, Alex, and I prank our friend Michael)*

Lean Health tells the story of how I went from having average health to having exceptional health in one year. I did it by applying my relentless application of making small incremental 2 second improvements. These small improvements of how I manage my health allowed me to develop the perfect system for me. This is what I achieved:

1. I lost 45 pounds. Most of my life I was over 210 pounds. Now I find it easy to maintain 165, which is the correct weight for my height of 5' 10".

2. The doctor says I look amazing and everything looks great when I go for a check up.

3. I have a strong, muscular body with a chiseled abdomen, something that was just a dream.

4. Finally and most important, I sustain exceptional health. After a full year of living healthy, I have no temptation to backslide into any

unhealthy habits. I just have a total love affair with serving and caring for my greatest customer…my body!

Most people want this for themselves but do not know how to get it. This book will lay out exactly what I did and give you the process I followed. You will see how I applied and think about lean ideas in every element of my life. Through my own personal stories and stories of others, you will learn to implement this simple Lean Health program, so you too can have exceptional health.

This book is also the story of how truly great friends can transform your life if you're willing to listen, collaborate and improve relentlessly. I stopped making the endless excuses of why I couldn't have excellence in every facet of my life. If we can be receptive to other people's ideas and not limit ourselves with negative self-talk, we can all accomplish much more than we ever thought possible. Excellent health is clearly within reach.

The One Thing:
You're Capable of way more than you ever dreamed

2secondlean.com/lh-01

Chapter 2

The Answer

There is no question that I'm an unorthodox person, so instead of making you wait until the end of the book for the key on how I achieved excellent health, I'm going to give it to you in this chapter. I'm doing this because I read a book recently that I really enjoyed, called "Overworked and Overwhelmed" by Scott Eblin. At the end of his book, Eblin summarized the entire thing by saying that it boils down to one word: breathe. Learn to breathe, he says, and your life will improve. This one-word summary makes it easy to remember Eblin's main point and how to implement his advice.

In the spirit of continuous improvement, wanting to be as clear as possible, I'm going to be straightforward and put my "answer" at the beginning of the book. That way, if you like what you read, you can continue reading and learn how I came to my conclusion. If you don't like it, you can put the book aside, email me and tell me you want a refund. I will be happy to send you one.

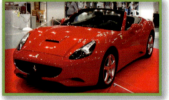
2014 Ferrari California
This is how I view my body

If I were going to summarize my entire book in one word it would be "Ferrari." The secret to excellent health—the answer—is to treat your body like you would treat a Ferrari. A Ferrari is the archetype of a sports car, one of the most precise and highest-performing machines ever made. It is exotic, fast, agile and beautiful. If you take the same care of your body that you would a Ferrari—using only the best fuel and regularly taking it to the best mechanic for maintenance—your body will return to you ten times what you put into it, for the duration of your life. Follow this principle, and you will make great strides in your own health.

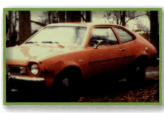
1974 Ford Pinto
This is how I used to view my body...anything goes

You can stop here, but if you want to learn more, keep reading. What follows is exactly what I do to maintain what I call Lean Health. It is a simple, straightforward method, with no

-16-

smoke and mirrors. I'm not a nutritionist, personal trainer, or health specialist. I'm just an average guy who figured out how to make his body perform at a very high level, and this is what I have done to get there. *(Go to the link at the end of this chapter to watch my video called How I Eat and How I Did It)*

Food and Drink

Eighty percent of my diet is fruits and vegetables and twenty percent is fish, chicken, cheese, nuts, and other types of protein.

When eating meat, I always look for fish first, because I like it the most and I feel best when eating it. Next, I look for chicken, which is still healthy, but perhaps not raised as naturally. Third, I eat pork, and fourth, beef. I am not against beef, I just do not feel as good when I eat it.

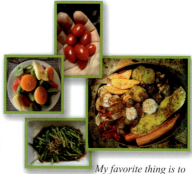

My favorite thing is to grab a handful of cherry tomatoes. Before Lean Health I ate them on my salads, now I eat them like candy

I eat nothing white—no flour, potatoes, bread, or sugar.

I avoid any processed foods (including breads, even if they are whole wheat). I want to eat things that come directly from the earth as much as possible, with a few exceptions (e.g., cheese, something I eat in moderation).

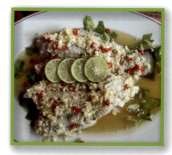

Thai Grilled Fish with Garlic and Red Peppers

I do not drink soda or consume artificial sweeteners. I relentlessly avoid anything processed.

All my cravings for sweets are satisfied with a delicious piece of fruit. My favorite piece of fruit is an apple, but I eat all kinds of exotic fruits from around the world and do not worry about the sugar content in them because the nutritional value of the entire fruit far outweighs any negatives from the

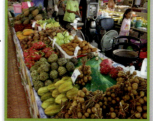

Market in Thailand

sugar. Again, these are only my opinions. I'm not a nutritionist, just a regular guy that achieved amazing health.

I log everything that goes into my mouth with the MyFitnessPal App so I know exactly what and how much I am eating. This is crucial to my success. I aim for exactly 2,400 calories each day, which is what my body needs to function at its highest level.

When I started logging my food, I learned I was eating way too much. To make matters worse, I was also logging lower quantities than I was actually eating. No longer!

Two tips to reduce your caloric intake: First, try using smaller plates. If you have to fit your food on a small plate or bowl, you are likely to eat less than you would if you used a large American-sized plate. Second, try using chopsticks. I have found that using chopsticks slows down my eating. These ideas are the result of making small 2 second improvements to the process to achieve excellent health.

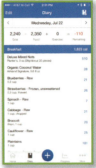

I log everything immediately after I eat it ... or you will forget

Regarding alcohol, I try to make every decision regarding what I put in my body based first on the health benefits and then on the taste. Fortunately, I've learned that the tastiest things are often the healthiest things. For example, the complexity of a beautiful red wine is matched with potential health benefits, so I regularly enjoy a glass with dinner. I like beer, but I generally stay away from it because the health effects do not match the satisfaction of the taste. This doesn't mean you can't drink beer—it just means I personally don't drink it much. For all other alcohol, I'll let you determine which to drink and which not to. Whatever you choose, remember to drink in moderation. As far as non-alcoholic drinks go I drink black tea, green tea, and black coffee. I also love soda water.

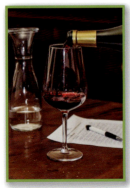

I drink one glass of red wine a day

Exercise

100 push-ups a day

100 sit-ups

100 trunk twists

Walk a minimum of 10,000 steps each day.

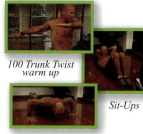
100 Trunk Twist warm up

Sit-Ups

Push-Ups

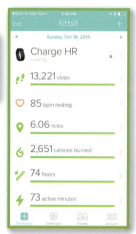
Minimum 10,000 steps

Psychology

The key is to love good foods and to hate bad foods. I have fallen in love with fresh vegetables and fruit.

I have a visceral disdain for anything processed. In my mind, processed food is poison. It might sound extreme, but it works perfectly and I have people all over the world following what I'm doing with the same success. I view my body as an amazing gift that I need to take care of with great care. When I look at myself in the mirror I see a Ferrari. I see a beautiful body that is giving me incredible satisfaction because I take care of it.

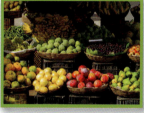
Pure health eat this if you want to be ripped and happy

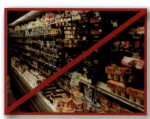
Poison...eat this if you want to be fat and sloppy

When I am honest with myself, I do not "self-deceive." When I am honest with myself about the need to monitor the quantity and the quality of what I eat, amazing things will happen. Facing this reality does not discourage me, it only sharpens my resolve and delivers better results.

Supplements

I take nothing—no vitamins, no aspirin, no steroids, no painkillers, and no sleep aids. I used to take most of these things but I have progressively weaned myself off of them and the result is my health is exceptional. This was not easy, but I believe our bodies are like pharmaceutical factories and can produce everything we need if we take care of them properly. I used to add protein powder to my smoothies, but now I add nuts instead.

You might be wondering right now what I did differently to have success where so many people have tried and failed. My best explanation is this: I took some of the Lean principles we use at my company, where we have great results and rarely produce defects, and started implementing them with my health.

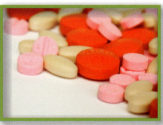

I cringe when I think of the things I have taken over the course of my life . . . NO MORE!

The fundamental idea behind Lean is continuous improvement through the elimination of waste. In order to expose waste, Lean practitioners look for it using the following categories. I have translated the classic wastes of Lean in the manufacturing world to how I see waste in the health domain.

1. Overproduction – We produce and consume too much food. Our bodies only need a fraction of the food we produce around the world, and much of the food we do produce is of poor quality, so we are overproducing poor-quality food that has very little nutritional value and a deleterious effect on our health.

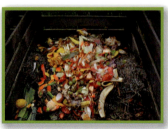

We make and eat way more than we need

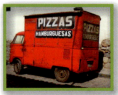

2. Transportation – We waste ridiculous amounts of energy transporting food all over the world, then we end up putting a huge percentage of the food in landfills because we can't even eat what we've transported (the irony is that we've already eaten 50% more than we needed in the first place). Transportation waste in the food system is staggering.

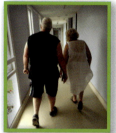

3. Inventory – We keep too much food inventory in our refrigerators, cupboards, and storage systems. However the worst form of inventory is the extra rolls of fat hanging off of most of us. All this fat creates mountains of defects in our health.

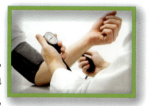

4. Defects – These include poor health, high blood-pressure, high cholesterol, a shorter lifespan, inactivity, poor self-esteem, indigestion, gas (too much bad food makes you fart!), and many others. Another defect is the poor example we set for our families and others (not the farting, but by our overall lackluster condition).

5. Over-Processing – Our medical system is forced to deal with

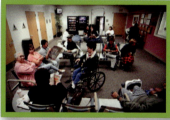

mountains of defects from obesity and obesity-related illnesses (diabetes, heart disease, etc.) We are applying ridiculous amounts of resources to solve problems that would be almost completely eradicated if we quit overproducing.

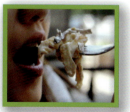

6. Excess Motion – We are lifting the fork to our mouths 75% more than is needed.

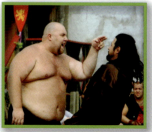

7. Waiting – The customer, our body, is waiting and waiting, hoping that someday we might listen to it and feed it high-quality food in the right quantity so it can perform the way it was intended.

8. Wasted Human Potential – The potential of our human bodies is remarkable, yet it is largely smothered and deeply muted because we have neglected to respect our bodies. The amazing gift each one of us has is dying to serve us at a very high level, but it cannot because of what we are sending down our throats every day.

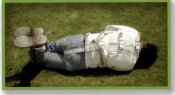
Wasted human potential

In the Lean process, waste is defined as anything the customer does not need or is not willing to pay for. In this case, your body is the customer and you are responsible for respecting it, nurturing it and feeding it properly. The body needs the proper amount of healthy, nutritious food, but most people overfeed it and give it poor quality food day in and day out. This produces fat, which actually decreases value and makes everything more difficult for our customer!

What we need to do is give our customer (our amazing body) exactly what it needs and stop pushing so much poor-quality products through its systems. When we eat or drink poorly, we create a lot of inconsistency in how we feel.

The variation in our results is both discouraging and unhelpful, so we want to eliminate it and make consistent improvements. To reduce variation, one of the Lean techniques we use is the standardization of processes. With Lean, you create very clearly defined processes by which you perform tasks. You perform an operation the same way every time until you create a better way of doing it. By doing this, you build repeatability and quality into the product.

One clearly defined process I use with my health is to start every day by consuming lots of vegetables. Every day, before the sun comes up, I make a large green smoothie for myself, starting with voluminous amounts of vegetables. I don't wait to get them in the afternoon with my salad or in the evening on my dinner plate. I begin consuming them from the second I get up. When I travel, it is not always practical to make a smoothie, so when I go looking for breakfast at the hotel or at a restaurant, my main goal is to find whatever vegetables and fruits I can. I always start with those.

In order to understand the effects of what we are consuming, we need good data. There is a famous quote about data that I love: "In

God we trust. Everyone else bring data." If you try to run your system without knowing what and how you are doing, it will fail. For my health, I log everything I eat on the MyFitnessPal App and monitor the number of steps I take with my FitBit. Now I know for sure when I am hitting my daily goal of 2,400 calories and 10,000 steps. When you record what you consume and how much you move, you know where you need to make improvements. You will begin to understand why variations are occurring and what adjustments you need to make to remove them. As you see your success, you are encouraged and want to be more disciplined in how you eat and exercise. The results speak for themselves.

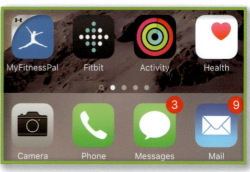

The most important Apps on my phone are in the most important position

Someone once said to me, "Paul you're a machine. I never met anybody with your level of discipline!" I paused and thought to myself, "Yes, I'm also red, have a six-hundred horsepower engine, and every detail has been hand-crafted to perfection...I'm a Ferrari in every aspect. And I enjoy the fact that everybody wants what I have!" I am able to maintain a high level of discipline and consistency because the results are ten times the effort that I'm putting into it.

People always ask me if I am tempted to eat some not-so-good food every once in a while. The truth is: No. Never. To me, the food I eat is the equivalent of driving a high performance Ferrari, while a piece of chocolate cake is a smoking Ford Pinto. There is no temptation. Lean Health works so well because it resolves the core problem. It educates and trains your brain about quality. It fundamentally changes your attitude and approach toward food. You no longer have to wrestle with your brain to make good decisions because it is now 100% aligned with your heart and emotions.

When I am honest with myself, I do not "self-deceive." When I focus on the quantity and the quality of what I eat, amazing things happen. Facing this reality does not discourage me, it only sharpens my resolve and delivers better results.

At 55-years-old, I know I can outperform 95% of all 18-year-olds because I'm committed to the quality food and exercise program that guarantees my health will be remarkable. However, Lean Health goes beyond just what I can achieve today, it is focused on long-term thinking. For me, that means I'm going to be vital and active for the rest of my life. In fact, I visualize myself skiing down the slopes of Aspen at 100-years-old!

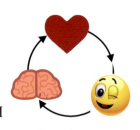

You no longer have to wrestle with your brain, your heart and emotions are 100% aligned with achieving excellent health

I view my body as an amazing gift that I need to take care of with great care. When I look at myself in the mirror, now I see a Ferrari. I see a beautiful body that is giving me incredible satisfaction because I take care of it.

The One Thing:
I am a Ferrari, not a Pinto

2secondlean.com/lh-02

Chapter 3

Everest Base Camp

As I begin to write this book, I have to confess something. I am going to talk about a subject that is probably the most important thing in my life improving, my personal health (and also bettering the lives of others). Nothing I've ever done has had a larger impact on my psychology, my personality, my well-being, and my overall disposition in life than this topic.

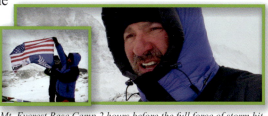

Mt. Everest Base Camp 2 hours before the full force of storm hit

In 2014, I was climbing up to Everest Base Camp on the slopes of the world's tallest mountain. *(Go to the link at the end of this chapter to watch my video on Everest Base Camp)* One of the largest storms in the last hundred years had just closed in on the Himalayas, and I was fortunate enough to make it to Base Camp at the last minute, just before the blizzard became so unbearable that

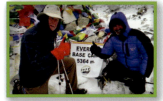

Dana and I at Base Camp 17,598 feet

nobody could return. It was about six o'clock when I stumbled into a tea house where I would spend the night freezing cold. I sat around the fire with about thirty other people, all trying to stay warm and feeling thankful we had shelter. The storm was so intense, it was blowing snow through closed windows, and the wind was blowing down the stove pipe and filling the main room with smoke from the yak dung burning stoves.

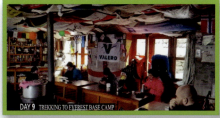

Gorokshep Tea House . . .It was one cold night

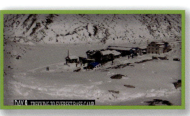

The day after the storm

The next day we began to understand what had transpired. The sun

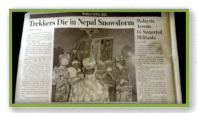
In Kathmandu we got the bad news

was out and it was a beautiful morning, but the Himalayas were blanketed with a couple feet of new snow. Hikers who normally came to this area to enjoy the beautiful terrain were now dealing with avalanches on all the passes. By the end of the day, we would learn that nearly 50 people had died in the previous day's storm. We were fortunate just to be alive.

I was exhausted and knew one thing for sure, I'd just spent the last eight days getting up to Base Camp and there was no way I was going to try to climb back down the mountain.

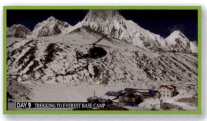
Helicopter landing in Gorokshep 16,863 feet coming to rescue us after the strom

It took me the rest of the day to secure a helicopter to fly up the mountain and retrieve our three-person group; my friend Dana, myself, and our guide. I will never forget the feeling of seeing that helicopter flying up the center of the valley knowing it was coming to rescue us.

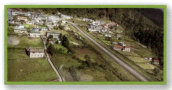
On short final, landing up hill into the side of the mountain

After riding the helicopter to the foot of the mountain, I turned on my phone to check my messages. I received an email from Audible, the audio book company, and opened it right away. Throughout my life, I had made it my discipline to read one book a week. I was constantly learning, growing, and extracting information from brilliant people around the world who shared what they had learned in their books.

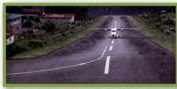
Downloading my emails in Lukla

Audible suggested I read a book called "Eat Move Sleep" by Tom Rath. I wasn't really interested in reading another health book. I'd read many other health books in my life, trying hard to implement the things I learned in them, but it was rare that any of them brought me significant results. I much preferred history books, historical novels, biographies, and books about current technology. Still, with a long trip ahead of me, I figured there was nothing to lose by giving it a try.

My friend Dana and I had decided to go to Thailand for a couple weeks, to recover and get warm, because we were so tired of from being cold after we summited Mount Kilimanjaro and Everest Base Camp back-to-back. I clicked download and shortly thereafter boarded a plane flying from Kathmandu to Phuket. *(Go to the link at the end of this chapter to watch my video on Mt. Kilimanjaro)* I spent the trip listening to the book and when I got to Thailand I was riveted by what I had learned during the flight. I was ready to get started on improving my health and transforming my life.

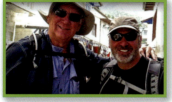
Dana and I on the first day of our trip

In his book, Rath writes that there are three things you need to do to have superior health: You need to eat quality food, you need to move at least 10,000 steps a day, and you need to sleep 8 hours a night.

I decided to start with his recommendations about movement. Up to this point in my life, I had never measured how much I exercised. I would go out and run on the treadmill for twenty or thirty minutes, but I never knew quantitatively what that meant in terms of my movement. Now for the first time, I would learn. I downloaded an App to my phone that told me how much I was moving every day. I made it a point to go out to the beach and walk and walk and walk, until I was hitting a consistent 10,000 steps a day. It seemed like a lot, but I was doing it! I always took the steps and avoided all elevators.

Next, I changed my eating habits. I cut out all the white flour, sugar, and artificial sweeteners from my diet and started focusing on eating fruits and vegetables. I only put into my body what was natural and avoided all processed foods. For breakfast, I no longer instinctively picked up a yogurt, pulled off the lid and ate it. Instead, I began to eat things like papayas, watermelons, and omelets, with some cheese on top, but nothing packaged.

Finally, I focused on sleep. In the past, if I was lucky, I would sleep two to three hours a night. After reading the book, I realized I needed to focus on going to bed at 9 o'clock so that I could wake up at 5 o'clock in the morning after having slept for 8 hours. While I didn't always make it to 8 hours, I did go from getting 2-3 hours of sleep per night to 5-6. This

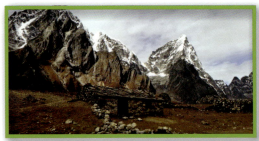
The best picture I have ever taken, in route to base camp

was a significant change for me, because now for the first time, my body was getting the rest it needed.

The results of these small improvements were remarkable, and they went way beyond just losing weight. They led me to create a system to achieve remarkable health that is simple and easy to follow.

For the last 15 years, using Lean principles to guide continuous improvement in manufacturing processes has been my passion. We should not try to confine Lean to the workplace, it can also greatly improve your home, personal life, and health.

Managing your health is a process no different than any other process. If you want to improve it, you must come up with a plan, run an experiment, evaluate the result, make adjustments, and then rerun the experiment. Doing this continuously, eliminating the non-value activity, delivering more value with each improvement cycle is the essence of continuous improvement.

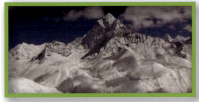
Flying out through the Himalayas the day after the storm

For example, I did not understand the detrimental effects that processed foods were having on my health. It did not matter how much I was exercising because as long as I was consuming so much processed food, I was not going to get the results I wanted. My first process improvement was eliminating processed foods from my diet, believing that would improve my health. I ran the experiment, and it worked. My weight came down and my overall health improved significantly. As soon as I was honest with myself about the types of foods I was eating, things began to improve. The simple system I created, based on these results, is what we are going to talk about in this book.

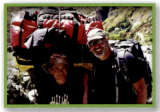
Our shurpa, half our size, carring our gear

Before moving onto the next chapter, I think it's appropriate that people understand philosophically how I think about life—why I go on all these adventures, why I do the things I do. I spent most of my life working extremely hard, always putting work first and play second. But when I turned 45-years-old, I realized I had been working so hard that I was in danger of allowing life to pass me by. I sat down, wrote out a bucket list and set about doing the things on it. I created my own radio show. I flew across the North Atlantic three times in a single-engine aircraft. I climbed mountains on several continents.

For the last ten years of my life, these adventures have been constant and consistent. I undertake them because life is short. We never know what tomorrow is going to bring, so I treat every day as if it's an adventure, as if I were a small child who is incredibly curious about what he can learn everywhere he goes in life.

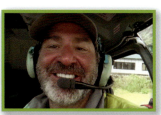
Happy day landing in Lukla

Today, as I write this book, I've been to almost 60 countries, every state in the United States, and almost every national park. I've done so many amazing things that most people wonder how in the world I've done so many. Recently, I was with Bob Taylor and he reached over and pinched my leg and described me as an "experience mosquito," looking for somewhere to land to extract an experience to make my life more full and rich. There is no better way to illustrate how I think.

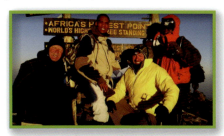
Dana and I on top of Mt. Kilimanjaro

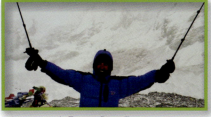
At Everest Base Camp

I succeeded by being deliberate about getting things done. I didn't say, "I'll do it next year." Starting when I was 45, I began to take lengthy trips multiple times every year. I started with one-week trips, then progressed to two weeks, then three weeks, and before long, the average trip for me was six weeks. The trip I'm on right now, as I'm writing this book, is two months long.

The truth of the matter is, you can do anything you want in life if you are deliberate about it. I cannot overemphasize the importance of deliberateness. I don't just allow things to happen by themselves. I plan them and make them happen. I develop habits that create the conditions for them to happen. And with that philosophy, I've been able to enjoy some of the most incredible things in life.

In spite of all these successes, though, there was one thing that had eluded me for years—having excellent health...but no longer! I'm excited to share all the things I've learned in life, whether it be my adventuresome spirit, my philosophy about running my company with Lean practices and now, Lean Health. My personal goal in life is to help people and encourage them to uncover their full potential. Every time I reach deep inside and attain a new height in my life, I am so delighted and excited about the discovery. My hope is that I can help other people feel the same thing that I feel...my potential is boundless and so is yours!

> ### THE ONE THING:
> EVEN THOUGH I WAS IN GOOD SHAPE, I HAD NO CLUE WHAT EXCELLENT HEALTH REALLY LOOKED LIKE

2secondlean.com/lh-03

Chapter 4

The Results

So, there I was in Phuket, Thailand, a place I'd never been before, but one I will never forget. The island's white sand beaches and turquoise waters make it one of the most beautiful places on Earth and one of the places I most enjoy visiting. *(Go to the link at the end of this chapter to watch my video on Phuket)*

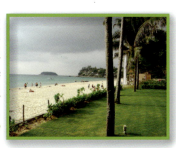

I spent the first week there dramatically changing how I moved, ate, and slept. I moved more 10,000 steps every day, period. The goal was non-negotiable. I had to do it. I ate better—only fresh fruits and vegetables, fish and chicken, nothing packaged, no sweeteners, and no sugars. If it grew out of the earth, it could go in my mouth, otherwise I wasn't interested. And lastly, I slept more. Five to six hours a day, compared to the 2-3 restless hours in the past. I made sleep a priority.

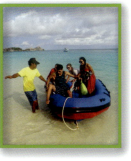

The results were surprising, even to me. When I came off of Everest Base Camp, right before flying to Thailand, I considered myself a very physically active person. Most people would look at me and tell me I was in good shape. In fact, I was in good shape (not great shape) but at the age of 54, I had just climbed Kilimanjaro's 19,500 feet, gone on a one-week safari, and travelled to Nepal to trek up to Everest Base Camp. Even after all this, I could still see the impact my new lifestyle had on my health. In one week, I went from 219 pounds (I'm five feet, ten inches tall) to 213 pounds. I lost 6 pounds in one week.

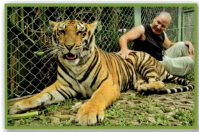

This is a photo of me at the beginning of my Lean Health journey

You might think that losing 6 pounds in a week is too much, too fast, but I didn't do anything crazy to make it happen. I just followed a simple, holistic concept that delivered fantastic results. Looking in the mirror, I immediately noticed some changes. I didn't look great yet, but I looked different, and it energized me.

The results indicated I was doing the right thing, and I wanted to do more. Positive results provide strong psychological reinforcement to continue working toward what we are trying to accomplish. When there are no results, or the results are marginal, it is difficult to stick with anything, but when you do something correctly and thoughtfully, the results will be there.

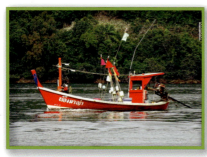

After one more week in Phuket, I left another few pounds lighter. I believed I had finally found a system that was going to work, something I could stick with that would help me achieve my health goals.

Others noticed the differences too. When I got home and walked into my company, my engineer, Dennis, said to me, "Oh, you got all skinny on us!" I don't know that I had ever heard anybody say those words to me. I've never been a skinny person in my entire life. I've always been a big-boned, Colorado farm boy, someone who had a little bit of meat on him, a fair amount of muscle, and a strength that said I shouldn't be messed with.

But Dennis' words shocked me. They triggered something in my brain I'd never felt before. For the first time, I believed I could attain a high level of physical fitness. I can do this, I thought. This can happen! The encouragement kept coming. Not a day went by when someone didn't say to me, "You look fantastic—wow! You're looking better and better and better!"

These words encouraged me to continue on the new path I had started in Phuket. It is amazing how just a few simple words can change your mind-set so dramatically. I think this is an important point. If words were powerful motivators for me, it is equally important that we are supportive of others. If you see somebody else embark on a Lean Health journey, make sure you support them and encourage them. Their journey could be life-changing as well, and you have the power to help them reach their goals.

> **THE ONE THING:**
> OPEN YOUR MOUTH AND ENCOURAGE SOMEONE...IT COULD CHANGE THEIR LIFE
>
> 2secondlean.com/lh-04

Chapter 5

How Could I Be So Stupid?

I consider myself relatively intelligent (not a Rhodes Scholar or a brain surgeon) but capable of consistently delivering common sense answers to problems in the sphere of my own life. However, the ability to consistently lose weight, keep it off and be in excellent physical health had always eluded me. For years, I struggled to understand why; was it my DNA that wouldn't allow me to achieve it? Or was it my stupidity?

Unfortunately, I found out on my journey to Thailand that my struggles had nothing to do with my DNA, and indeed, were caused by my stupidity. Thanks to Tom Rath's book, I learned it only took three things—deliberately moving more (i.e., taking 10,000 steps a day), eating foods that were not packaged and processed, and sleeping 8 hours a night to deliver the results I was looking for. Today, I can only laugh at myself because I'm 55-years-old, college-educated and extremely successful and it still took me this long to figure out the secret to being healthy.

Looking back, I can't understand how I missed the answer for so long. It was so simple and obvious! Yet the important thing is that now I understand and want to let as many people know that having excellent health (exceptional health, rather) is completely and totally attainable.

This book is called Lean Health, and its purpose is to show you how applying Lean principles in your life can help you reach your health goals. At its most fundamental level, Lean is about continuous improvement. I regularly looked for ways to lose weight and improve my physical shape. A few times each year, I would go on a different diet, but I was never able lose weight consistently. I stayed about the same and kept repeating my ineffective habits.

The worst part was that I accepted the results, even though I wasn't making progress. I told myself, oh well, that's just who I am. This was my biggest mistake. We can say that something is "just who we are," but this acceptance of mediocrity is the main problem. Telling myself that I could not get better is where my stupidity showed itself.

The moment we accept mediocrity or accept the status quo is the moment we become stupid. How could a human being, with all our capacity and sophistication (a skeletal system, a circulatory system, a nervous system, a brain, a heart and emotions) ever accept mediocrity?

The irony is using our intelligence to become more healthy is easier, simpler and more enjoyable than being unhealthy. Everything about being healthy is better. We sometimes rationalize not being healthy because we think it's a lot of work, but it is actually less work! This is the staggering revelation I've come to after 55 years on Earth. When I eat healthy, I always feel good. When I eat healthy, I have no ups and downs. When I eat healthy, my body loves me and rewards me with emotional energy that I've never had before. Everything about eating correctly, exercising and respecting your body is better, easier, simpler and makes your life more full. I was so stupid to take this long to figure out something that was right in front of my face.

The analogy I like to use to understand the importance of being healthy is this: people's bodies are like airplanes; they work best when they are not overweight. I'm a pilot, and I know that if a plane is overweight, it doesn't fly well, it's out of balance and the controls are difficult to handle. When you take off in a plane, you have just what you need and no more. You carry extra fuel, but only enough to fly an additional hour in case you need to get to a nearby airport for an emergency.

Our bodies work the same way. It is best when they do not carry a lot of extra fuel (fat). However, most people carry not just an extra hour's worth of fuel, or a day's worth of fuel, or even a week's worth of fuel. We walk around with months of fuel weighing us down. This is craziness! Could you imagine taking off in a plane with enough fuel to fly around the world when you're only going on an hour-long trip?

How much bigger would the airplane have to be to support all this extra fuel? It would have to fly more slowly while expending a lot more energy and creating more wear on the plane's engines, just to carry the excess weight of the fuel.

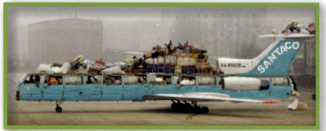

If you think this looks stupid, you should take a good look at what we are putting in our bodies

This is exactly what we do to our bodies when we carry around so much extra weight. We move more slowly, expend more energy and add extra stress to our muscles, joints and organs. When we reduce that extra weight, our bodies function at optimum performance; we are faster, more agile and can navigate the world with less effort.

We deceive ourselves into thinking that somehow it's acceptable to go around with 30-40 extra pounds, believing we have no power to change. This is insanity and we must not allow ourselves to believe this deception. Once I figured out I was deceiving myself, it became much easier to change. I have completely shifted the way I view life, health and food. Now for me, an easy, quick snack is grabbing an apple and tasting it, knowing the good it's doing to my body. Picking up a tomato from the counter top, putting it in my mouth and tasting things I've never tasted before is more satisfying than processed foods and there is no downside. Eating becomes one hundred percent positivity from start to finish, something it doesn't take a brain surgeon to understand. You have no regrets and don't suffer the emotional drain that comes from eating junk food.

My good friend, Dana May, who is also doing Lean Health said, "People need to understand you're not giving up anything and it is totally a net gain in every regard in your life." The interesting thing about this comment from Dana is he is someone who used to have 3-4 drinks a night, eat all kinds of fried foods and sugary desserts and would often smoke a cigar in the evening. If anyone had to give something up to practice Lean Health, Dana would be the prime candidate. However, he feels like he is giving up nothing. I feel exactly the same way, and I've never felt this way about anything before. The positives are overwhelming!

> **THE ONE THING:**
> BEING HONEST WITH YOURSELF WILL ALWAYS PRODUCE A BETTER OUTCOME
>
> 2secondlean.com/lh-05

Chapter 6

We Are All Addicts

When I was 16-years-old, my high school woodshop teacher was John Pruitt. John was a good friend who mentored me as I became a woodworker. One day, he invited me out to lunch and as we were driving down the road in his truck, he popped open a diet soda and said, "Man, do I love this stuff!"

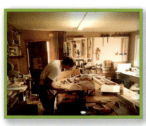

In my early years as a wood craftsman

I grimaced at him, questioning how anyone could like diet soda, but he assured me he was telling the truth. "Everybody's got a vice," he said. I've never forgotten him saying that, because at that moment, I realized he was right, everybody is some kind of addict. I also realized that food had become my addiction, something I used for the purpose of feeling good and was I ever a heavy user! A person of my size, at 5' 10", should consume about 2,400 calories per day. But I was eating 4,000 to 5,000 calories a day. I could easily put away a 1,000 calories in a single meal. Looking back, now I understand that food had become a drug for me, and the foods I was eating were actually causing me to want to eat more.

You might be skeptical. After all, I'm no scientist, I'm not a health or nutrition expert either. I'm just thinking back on what was happening in my own life. I was eating foods that created a craving (an addiction if you will) to eat more food. They weren't satisfying, so I just kept eating more and more. I would eat a bunch of refined carbohydrates and a short time later, I was hungry again and wanted more. I was also eating a lot of artificial sweeteners, and I'm convinced they had a detrimental effect on me. The science regarding the correlation between consuming artificial sweeteners and increased cravings for sweets is not definitive yet. At the very least, I loved food to the point that I was addicted to it. I always wanted it.

If the story ended there, it would be a sad one. However, things have changed in my life. Now I love food, but for entirely different reasons than before. I'm still an addict, but I'm addicted to healthy foods. My mind and body think about food entirely differently. I want food because it has this amazing, nourishing effect on my body. Everything about the human body is staggering. We have five finely-tuned senses. We have a complex brain that allow us to create things and solve problems that no other species can. Our bodies are like Ferraris, designed for great performance and amazing abilities. We can run, walk, and climb mountains. Nobody who has a car of that caliber would put cheap gas in it or take it to an average mechanic. You would treat it very special, just like you should treat your body.

This is my new perspective. I'm addicted to fantastic food that nourishes my own precision engine. The only thing I want to put in it is healthy foods: fruits, vegetables, fish (only top quality fuel for me). Every time I eat well, I have this amazing feeling come over me as if I am taking perfect care of my inner Ferrari.

Moreover, because I am taking good care of my body, I never feel ups and downs. Being a Lean practitioner, I know that large swings up and down are not good for productivity. In a manufacturing setting, we want evenness and consistency in everything we do. This produces the least amount of waste and ultimately produces the highest quality outcome with the fewest number of defects. My new addiction provides evenness and consistency to my physiological needs.

Eating healthy gives me a more even, consistent appetite. I wake up in the morning and I don't have the cravings I used to have. Sure, I want to eat, but not because my body is screaming "FEED ME!" Instead, it tells me (in a calm voice), "Hey, let's go nourish this amazing machine."

Recently, I was at a job site in Kazakhstan, in the middle of nowhere. One morning, I was working hard on a project and when lunchtime came around, I had not eaten in 4 hours. In the past, if I had not eaten for that long, I would be going crazy, thinking, I'm starving, I've got to eat! When the food would come, I would plow

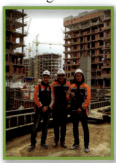
At job site in Kazakhstan

-39-

through it, eating so fast I could barely taste it.

Now, because I am addicted to healthy food, when it is time for lunch, I think, hey sure, let's go eat. I'm going to nourish my body. I am able to slow down and enjoy the food. I realize now my eating habits have changed because I have a fantastic new addiction to healthy food.

I never thought I would say I'm happy that I'm an addict, but I love my new addiction! I'm happy that I love food because I want it to nourish me and not because I need to gorge myself like some food maniac. If we all have to be addicted to something, why shouldn't it be fantastic, nourishing food that supports a healthy physiological outcome? I am proud to say that I am an addict of high-quality food and I am never going back to my old habits.

80% fruits and vegetables
20% chicken and fish

Falling in love with good food is probably the most important component to understanding Lean Health and moving to a high level of personal well-being. In the past, I've always enjoyed healthy foods, but I was never in love with them. Now I'm falling in love with food on two different levels; first, with the flavors; and second, with what it actually does to my body. It's an entirely different eating experience.

In the past, if I saw pastries sitting on a counter, I would grab one and eat it, almost without thinking. Today, my mind has so fundamentally changed from where it once was that when I walk past some pastries, I immediately think, that's the stuff that makes me fat. That's the stuff that makes me look like a slob!

Conversely, when I walk up to a counter with tomatoes, carrots, or beets on it—any kind of vegetable, I think, I've got to have that now! It is as if I have a love affair going on every time I see something natural that comes out of the ground. When I put a tomato in my mouth, not only does it taste wonderful, but I am also releasing vitamins and nutrients to supercharge my body and make it strong, fit, and lean, and that gets me excited!

The process excites others too. When I traveled to Kazakhstan for business, a man named Metin picked me up at the airport. When I got off the plane, he looked at me and said, "Wow, you look good!" 55-year-old men like me don't usually get compliments on how they look, but he said, "Man, you're ripped. You look amazing!"

"I know," I said. "It was so easy too. I feel so stupid that it took me so long to figure it out."

Metin asked me what I was doing to get in this kind of shape and I said, "You know, it's really quite simple. I just eliminated all the bad things out of my diet and focused on all the good things." More specifically, I told him, 80% of my diet is fruits and vegetables, with the balance being protein—fish, chicken, cheese, and nuts. I explained how I used to consume lots of artificial sweeteners, buying it by the bag full and adding it to every cup of tea and coffee I drank. The very stuff I believed was helping me stay thin (though I wasn't thin) was the exact thing making me fat.

As soon as I mentioned artificial sweeteners, a light came on in Metin's mind. "Wow, I'm addicted to diet soda," he exclaimed. "I've been drinking 3-4 of them every day for 40 years. I get out of bed and the first thing I do is I drink it."

I said, "Metin, you will not believe what will happen to you if you wean yourself off of this stuff."

Without hesitation, he said, "I'll do it!"

Now, imagine a man who's been drinking this stuff constantly for 40 years, and all of a sudden says he is going to quit. You might be somewhat skeptical, but the next day when he picked me up, he said, "I did it. No more diet soda." For the two weeks I was in Kazakhstan, Metin did not drink any more diet soda. As we ate together, I watched him, and he began to focus on eating good foods. He began to eat fruits and vegetables, taking his first steps toward Lean Health.

In such a short time, had Metin broken his 40 year habit? Had his psychology completely changed in two weeks? Probably not, but he did take a powerful first step. He told me he now looks at diet soda as "the black poison." His words were a powerful insight into human psychology.

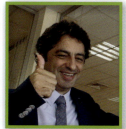

Metin breaking his 40 year habit of drinking diet soda "the black poison"

He had created a strongly negative mental image of the beverage to discourage himself from drinking it.

This is exactly what I do with my own diet. I look at the starches and all the cheap substitutes for real food in the world and think of them as poison. I look at them as the things that make people fat and sloppy. I don't stop there. I also fall in love with the good aspects of healthy food.

The beautiful thing about this strategy is that it is two-sided. On one side, you create negative associations with the bad foods (e.g., Metin calling diet soda "black poison") and on the other side, you fall in love with fruits and vegetables. With these 2 simple steps, you move your diet toward a healthy one that will completely change the way your body feels.

I'll share one other story that demonstrates some of the benefits of falling in love with good food. After two weeks in Kazakhstan, we had an executive meeting with all the top leaders of the company I was working with. At the start of the meeting, the president of the company said something that shocked me. He said, "You know, Paul is not just demonstrating Lean by the way he runs his company. He's not just telling us to run our company well, but he's also in good lean physical health. And I know because I saw him with his shirt off in the sauna. He's 55-years-old and he has ribs and he has a six pack." Then he looked around at his leadership team of eight people and said, "We haven't seen this since our mid-20s and early 30s. It's all gone. Paul sets a great example for us."

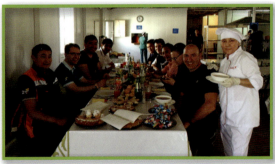

They prepared fruits, vegetables, and fish for me. The chef and staff went above and beyond to make sure I was happy.

Think about that for a moment. We were at the board meeting of a billion-dollar organization and the president was using my health as an example to be followed. That's what happens when you fall in love with good food!

In addition to eating right, exercise is extremely important to health too, and the technique of creating mind associations to change your behavior works with it as well. For example, when I see an elevator, I think of an elevator as a *death elevator* because it helps me become fat and sloppy. I always used to take the elevator because it was easier, but now I want to be lean, trim, and healthy and live to 100 (which is my goal), so I take the stairs instead.

The formula for great health is fairly simple. Reject negative food. Fall in love with good food. Create powerful connections in your mind that support the habits you want to have in your life and you will be successful.

> ## THE ONE THING:
> CREATE POWERFUL CONNECTIONS IN YOUR MIND

2secondlean.com/lh-06

Chapter 7

Never Sick

For whatever reason, I grew up with a weak immune system, and it seems like I spent my entire life in a recurring cycle of sickness. I would get sick for three weeks, then I'd get a little better, then I'd get sick again, and the next thing you know, I'd have to go back to the doctor for antibiotics. The antibiotics would heal me for a few weeks, but I would soon return to the tiresome routine of being sick.

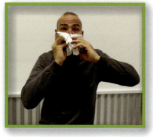
Always sick

One of the causes was the environment around me. I used to be a cabinetmaker, and I inhaled a lot of dust while I was working. In my mid-30s, I found out that all the dust was aggravating my sinuses, making me constantly sick. I used to improve my condition by doing a saline rinse, which requires you to snort warm salt water up your nose to rinse out your sinuses. It helped a lot, so I did it frequently, but I was still constantly sick.

As my company grew, I did less woodworking and more public speaking. During the winter, particularly when colds and flus were going around, I would carry a bag of cough drops with me to all my speaking engagements. About an hour before giving a speech, I would start sucking on them, to make sure my throat would be numb and I wouldn't be hacking and coughing in front of several hundred people. The drops calmed the symptoms, but they did nothing to keep me healthy. It always seemed like the minute I got within five feet of someone who was sick, I would get sick again. It was very frustrating because I wanted to be healthy, but I didn't know how.

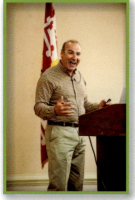
Sucking on my cough drops before my speeches

Then, something remarkable happened. In Thailand, after I started this new way of eating and taking care of myself, my friend Dana got sick. I was expecting to get sick myself, but I stayed healthy for the rest of our time in Thailand and then throughout the journey home. When I walked into my company where 50 employees, several of whom were sick, greeted me, I was certain my health would change for the worse. But it didn't!

To my surprise, I went another three months and remained healthy, even though it was the middle of the winter when everyone around me, including my wife, got sick. Over the next several months, I traveled around the world three times and went on more airplanes than you could shake a stick at. I shook the hands of hundreds of people at conferences and consulting gigs all over the world, and I still did not get sick.

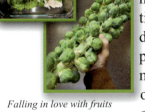

Falling in love with fruits and vegetables

Today, as I'm writing this chapter, nearly one year has passed since the last time I was sick. I asked myself why? What is different in my life that would create such a profound change in my wellness? The only thing I can think of is the change in my diet. I removed all artificial sweeteners and anything that was processed, and added voluminous amounts of fruits and vegetables, especially broccoli, a superfood.

These days, I eat a ton of broccoli. I buy large bags of pre-cut broccoli at Costco and put it in my smoothie every morning. I cook it for dinner at night. By the end of the day, I've probably eaten 4-5 cups of broccoli, more than most people eat in a month. I believe the broccoli and all the fruits and vegetables are supercharging my body so I never get sick.

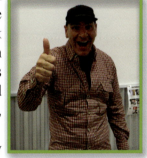

Never sick

Now, I'm sure that sooner or later I'm going to catch a cold or get the flu, but so far, I've stayed healthy. This is perhaps the greatest benefit of this new process for maintaining my health. I no longer have to waste so much time going to the doctor or taking antibiotics, so I have more time and energy to spend on being productive.

I do not want to sound like I am opposed to antibiotics or modern medicine. Not at all. I'm simply making the point that when you eat correctly, you generally don't need any additional supplements to be healthy. Once again, these are my opinions as a non-professional. I'm not a nutritionist or a physician, I'm just making simple observations. Why does this system work? There is a principle called Occam's Razor that may explain what is happening. Occam's Razor states that the solution to most things is the most obvious or simplest one. Regarding my health, the most obvious explanation is that consuming large amounts of fruits and vegetables has strengthened my immune system. A better diet, plus a consistent exercise regime, have given me exceptional health.

This new lifestyle has created such a powerful change in my overall well-being that I wouldn't trade where I am for anything. I am, to say the least, elated with the outcome.

THE ONE THING:
BROCCOLI RULES

2secondlean.com/lh-07

Chapter 8

The Four Things I learned from Doug

When I was about 2 1/2 months into my new health regime, I thought I was doing fantastic, but would soon learn otherwise. A good friend of mine, Doug Scoggins, the general contractor who built our company's new building, said I should come work out with him. Doug is an unusual individual. He

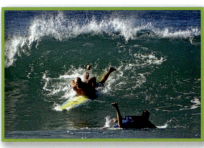

Fantastic surf in Costa Rica

runs a large construction company with lots of employees and he also maintains perfect physical health. Doug was a state champion in kick boxing, and in addition to being a contractor, he owns and operates a gym in Ferndale, Washington. When it comes to athleticism, he is at a level I have never seen anybody else reach. When you watch him work out, you are astounded at what he can do, whether he is doing pull-up after pull-up or effortlessly doing endless push-ups.

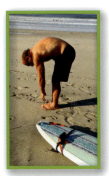

When Doug asked me to come to his gym at 5:15 a.m. to work-out with him and thirty other people, I hesitated. "I can barely get out of bed to work-out at my house, let alone go work-out with you," I told him. He persisted, so I went. I needed to get in shape anyway. I was preparing for another adventure, a month-long trip to Costa Rica to learn how to surf. To get ready for the trip, I had been working out at my home gym every day for 20-30 minutes, running

Early morning stretching on the treadmill or doing the rowing machine and lifting some weights. I thought I was getting into pretty good shape.

As it turns out, I had no clue what it meant to work-out. When I showed up at the gym that first morning, Doug kicked my ass. There is no other way to put it. I was wringing wet at the end of an hour. Doug pushed us through circuit after circuit, from boxing to burpees to pull-ups. We did 60 rounds of intense exercise with short breaks of 15-30 seconds in between. After about a week, I was addicted to the intensity, and I realized that if I trained this hard I would easily be in the physical shape to be able to master surfing and endure the pounding of the waves. *(Go to the link at the end of this chapter to watch my workout videos)*

Doug also knew I would be ready to surf, but he threw in another challenge. He said, "Paul, let's get you below 200 pounds." At this point, I was about 203 pounds, down from about 219 when I came down from Everest Base Camp. I was doing great but, I wanted so badly to get below the 200 pound mark. I told Doug I was struggling with my weight. He told me with total clarity and surety, "You're eating more than you think. You need to control your portion size." I'll never forget those words. It was then I realized that if I continued to work out with the same intensity and controlled my portion size, I would indeed drop below 200 pounds. In just another week, I had made it. *(Go to the link at the end of this chapter to watch my portion control videos)*

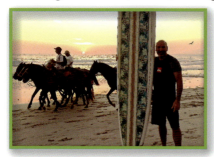
Surfing till sundown

To help me get there, Doug taught me how to get more vegetables in my diet. Up to this point, I was not drinking smoothies, but Doug said something very powerful to me. He said, "You can bury a lot of vegetables in a smoothie."

"What do you mean?" I asked.

"Every morning I wake up and I put spinach, broccoli and all kinds of vegetables in my smoothie," he explained. "Then I add blueberries, an apple, a banana, or strawberries. But I always start every smoothie with lots of vegetables."

I started to do the same thing and the results were incredible. I felt better about myself. I noticed my overall health and well-being improving. I lost more weight and sharpened my focus on what optimal health looked like. *(Go to the link at the end of*

Respect nature, the ocean is powerful

this chapter to watch my healthy eating videos)

A key lesson I learned from Doug was that we are very good at deceiving ourselves. I used to think I ate well, but I had no clue what eating well meant. I used to think I worked out hard, but I didn't know what that meant either. I convinced myself I was doing well, but looking at Doug's physique, I realized I was wrong. There was nothing in my life that suggested I was operating at a high level of fitness. I had deceived myself into believing that the moderate approach to my diet and exercise would someday help me achieve exceptional health. This was a huge deception. Now, instead of doing things halfheartedly, I realized I needed to workout with deliberateness and intensity, and I needed to monitor both the quality and quantity of what I put into my body. If I could do that, the results would be amazing.

Once I learned those lessons well, Doug told me one more thing that completely blew me away. As my body changed and my physique improved, he said, "Paul you're **aging in reverse**. You're actually getting younger." As I reflected on what he was telling me, I knew he was right. If you take care of yourself properly, you can **age in reverse**. I feel like I'm 18-years-old again and there is nothing I can't do.

Three months into my Lean Health journey. Looking and feeling better

As a matter of fact, when I'm home at my company's facility, after we finish our morning meeting and our stretching, we have a push-up challenge. All of us get down and see how many push-ups we can do until we're exhausted. I have a lot of young studs that work for me, but no one can beat me. Once or twice somebody did beat me, but only because they were cheating. When we had someone make sure everybody was doing the push-ups the same way, they couldn't keep up. Imagine, a 55-year-old man who can do more push-ups than fit 18-year-olds and 22-year-olds. Thanks to Doug, this was no accident.

Ultimately, Doug taught me there is no excuse for not working out. He sets the best example because he is a successful businessman with a large company, yet he makes no excuses for why he cannot take incredible care of his body. He is my inspiration for bringing it to the next level and frankly why I look the way I do. Today, not a single day goes by without me thinking about Doug and what he can do.

As for the surfing, I did go to Costa Rica and learn how to surf. In fact, I was very successful at it, and I credit a lot of my success to Doug and the lessons he taught me

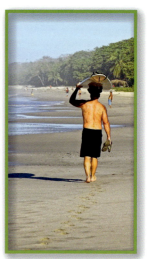

The One Thing:
Listen to the voice of success

2secondlean.com/lh-08

Chapter 9

Convoluted Chemistry

Our culture has introduced many new compounds into the diet via processed and packaged foods. We commonly eat processed breads, meats, or even meals that have lists of ingredients that are ten, twenty, sometimes thirty items long. The body takes this stuff in and says, "What do I do with this? I wasn't made to work with this. I'll just put it over here to store in my fat cells."

In my opinion, the body works best when it is in a totally natural state, ingesting foods that are nutritious and provide all the necessary vitamins and minerals it needs to function efficiently. This is not how most people in western society eat. They have convoluted the chemistry of their bodies by eating these processed foods. This is exactly what I was doing prior to my Lean Health discovery.

Next, we complicate things further by taking an endless array of over-the-counter and prescription drugs. You might not believe me, but I challenge you to find anyone that doesn't take some kind of medication. When I go to the doctor and they ask me, "Do you have any allergies? Do you have resistance to any drugs? Do you take anything?" I tell them I have no allergies and I take nothing. When I say this, they look at me in disbelief. "What! You don't take anything?" This is such a foreign concept these days. Everybody is taking something to regulate something, and this convolutes the chemistry occurring inside our bodies.

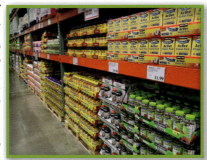

Hard to believe that we have been told to take these, when all you need to do is eat healthy

In the Lean world, we call this over-processing. We have overwhelmed our body's functions by adding all this unnecessary garbage to our bodies. The net result is a confused and convoluted chemistry and a body that does not function like it should. Again, these are all just my own personal observations and conclusions, using my common sense.

In an earlier chapter, I talked about Occam's Razor; the idea that the most logical answer is the one that's right in front of you. If you look at all the health problems that exist in Western society, you have to ask yourself what the most obvious common denominators are. I say diet and drugs, or what I call the DD factor. We are overdosing on the DD factor. We are convoluting our natural chemistry. The more I have weaned myself off these foreign substances, the better I feel. I marvel every time I go to the doctor for a check-up and they look at me and say, "How could anybody at 55-years-old look like you and have the health makeup you have? We don't see this." I tell them it is very simple. I'm careful about what I eat, I exercise regularly, and I treat my body like a Ferrari. It is just common sense.

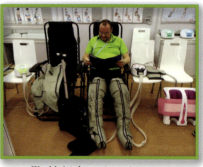
Wouldn't it be easier to just get up, exercise and eat quality food?

I haven't always had this common sense. I only learned it over the course of the last year and that is why I'm writing this book. I want to share as much as I can with other people in hopes that they can dramatically improve the quality of their lives through the application of simple common sense ideas and a profound process that I call Lean Health. You don't have to over-process your life. The next time your body is reacting strangely to something, or you don't feel good, ask yourself this question, "Am I in some way convoluting the chemistry inside me?" If you are, think about how you can get it back to that natural, fully-functioning state by reducing your dependence on processed foods and different types of drugs.

THE ONE THING:
DON'T CONVOLUTE THE CHEMISTRY

2secondlean.com/lh-09

Chapter 10

Traveling is Easy

One of my favorite sayings is, "If you don't ask, the answer is always no. If you just ask, you'll be surprised how often the answer is yes." I have learned this applies to traveling as well. Sticking to a health regimen or particular way of eating while traveling can be especially challenging, but it doesn't have to be. I've learned some powerful lessons about how to be more faithful to our bodies on the road, and it started with a story in Tom Rath's book, "Eat Move Sleep." Rath says that when he goes to a restaurant, the worst temptation comes at the end of the meal when the waiter asks if he wants dessert. At this point, many people lose their discipline. They indulge in a dessert that adds a few hundred unnecessary (and unhealthy) calories to the meal. Rath explains how he treats himself to dessert, but in a healthier way. He says that most restaurants always have some kind of fresh fruit available, even if it's not on the menu. All you need to do is ask. I immediately latched on to this concept and whenever I feel like I want something special after a meal, but don't want to wreck my diet, I ask if I can have some fruit. It almost always works. Most restaurants enjoy trying to please their customers.

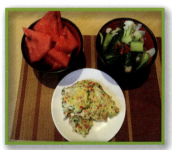
Breakfast in China

You might be surprised to find out how accommodating people will be to dietary requests. On my recent trip to Kazakhstan, a place off the beaten path for most Westerners, I told my hosts when I arrived that I am very careful about what I eat and if possible, I would only like to eat fruits, vegetables, fish and chicken. Not only were they accommodating, but they seemed to go out of their way just to please me. I think they got as much pleasure out of seeing me satisfied

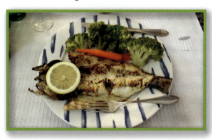
Dinner in Thailand, hold the rice please. Fresh grilled fish and broccoli. It's never on the menu, you just have to ask

as I got from maintaining my healthy lifestyle. It didn't matter where I went, everyone knew it was fruits, vegetables, fish and chicken for Paul. I didn't feel like I put my hosts out. As a matter of fact, just the opposite. They loved the concept of accommodating my simple way of eating.

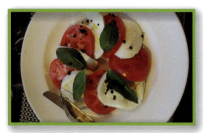
No excuses, there is always a good option

Sometimes, it takes a little extra effort to maintain the regimen. Being at the airport can be bad for your health because every convenience store or fast food place is full of packaged food. Our society is set up around packaged or processed products, but it is still possible to find the things you need if you turn on your eyes. For instance, when I was in the Bangkok Airport, all the stores sold junk food, but I knew there was one thing I could eat that would maintain my health and nourish my Ferrari body, nuts. I searched from one store to another until finally I found a store that sold a bag of mixed nuts. I bought a couple and instead of blowing my diet (even though I don't consider this a diet, it's a lifestyle), I enjoyed and savored every bite, knowing I was eating real food.

Later, when it was time to eat a full meal, all I saw were fast food restaurants everywhere, from Dairy Queen to Burger King to KFC. I knew it was highly unlikely any of them would have the food I was looking for. Among all the fast food places, though, I noticed one Thai restaurant that looked like it made fresh food. The menu did have a lot of fried food, noodles and other things that I did not want, so I asked if they had any salmon. They said yes. I asked if they had broccoli. They did. Could they make me salmon with broccoli? They said yes to that, too. Eight minutes later, my plate arrived with a beautiful piece of fresh salmon, right there in the middle of a fast food court. They only gave me one sprig of broccoli and two baby corns, a little bit of sweet potato and one carrot slice, so I asked for a little more. Four minutes later, they

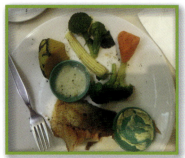
Eating healthy in Bangkok airport

brought me a plate of fresh steamed broccoli. In the middle of the most unlikely place in the Bangkok Airport, I was eating perfectly, just as I wanted. It is really amazing what happens when you are determined to take care of yourself. *(Go to the link at the end of this chapter to watch my travel videos)*

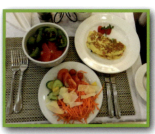
Breakfast, nothing packaged, just nourishing my Ferrari and enjoying the taste of fresh foods

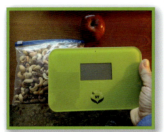
Three essentials I never leave home without to guarantee I stay in exceptional health. Apple, unsalted nut mix, and travel scale.

Often when we embark on anything of substance, it is easy to make excuses for why we won't succeed, but we have no time for excuses. They don't do anything for us except perpetuate our own self-deception. Another favorite saying of mine is, "Life is not a rehearsal." Each day is not a practice for the "real" day ahead. Each one is real right now, and we need to take advantage. There are no do-overs. Why not start taking care of your body now? Why not receive all the benefits of taking care of your body now? It doesn't matter where you are. You can maintain a consistent and healthy diet, even when you're on the road. Traveling is not so hard. Traveling is easy.

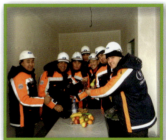
Even on the job site in Kazakhstan they had fresh fruit for me at break time ... I really think they enjoyed it as much as I did!

THE ONE THING:
JUST ASK...THE ANSWER IS USUALLY YES

2secondlean.com/lh-10

Chapter 11

The Big Deception

Throughout the past chapters you have heard me talk repeatedly about how we deceive ourselves. This concept came to me when I was about eight months into my new way of thinking about life and health. I was sitting in my kitchen and I suddenly thought, wow, I have totally deceived myself for the past 55 years!

Before my revelation, I used to tell myself one lie after another. When it came to my health, the biggest one was that genetically I wasn't made to be thin. I would tell myself that I was a Colorado farm boy and that my dad was a big guy who was overweight, my brother is overweight and I was overweight. It was just the way we rolled.

This is the type of self-deceptive talk I would hear constantly inside my head. If the negativity ended there, it would have been bad enough. But it did not, and I would further deceive myself, with thoughts like, "It's so difficult to eat right. It's so tempting to eat those pastries. Gosh! Why does my wife make all those good things that make me go off my diet? If only I was in charge of the grocery shopping, I would never have these problems. My kids bring home all that junk food. Every day at work somebody is bringing doughnuts. I go to conferences and they put a piece of chocolate cake in front of me. I was born with these disabilities and health problems and I have to medicate. I can't walk. My ankle hurts. I have to get up too early in the morning to exercise. Work is so stressful. I don't have an athletic body. I wasn't born like one of those skinny people who can eat anything and have no problems. My family loves to eat and I was expected to love food from the moment I came out of the womb. My dad always slapped me upside the head and told me to finish the food on my plate because there were people starving all over the world. I've been overeating since I was 6-years-old and there's no way I'm going to stop now. I just love sugary things. I'm addicted to chocolate. I can't stop myself.

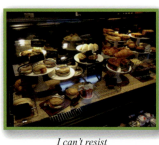
I can't resist

I eat one bite of pastry and then the next thing you know, I've devoured 4 of them. I love my coffee with tons of sweeteners and that mocha flavoring. I drive by coffee shops and an invisible lasso ropes me around the neck and pulls me in. There are only a few people in the world who are really skinny and everybody else is just a little overweight. It's good to carry some fat on you just in case you get sick. It doesn't matter that I'm overweight. I've learned to be happy with myself. All those pictures on the front of Men's Health magazine, they're all 'Photoshopped'. Those guys are all on steroids. There's no way you can look like that. They're just lucky they have bodies like that. The rest of us don't have it that good. My wife doesn't support me. She is a junk food addict. I love potato chips. I love that salty taste. I need that diet soda, it gets me going. That caffeine is something that I have to have.

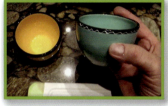
Try eating out of a small bowl

All those people who are skinny and proposed all those diets, they're just lucky and their body metabolizes things totally differently than the rest of us. Jack LaLanne, he's a fraud. Those people who are that skinny, it's all liposuction. They're all taking drugs. Thin-thin, win-win, din-din, who the hell knows, it's all drugs. That's the only way they could be so skinny!" I think you get the picture.

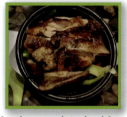
I took a normal size bowl form Panda Express with teriyaki chicken (no sauce) and vegetables. Chopped it up and filled three small bowls.

We are all pretty good at self-deception, aren't we? We feed ourselves a bunch of lies and excuses. I used to be the master of it too, but now I know better. I felt like an idiot that morning when I realized I had been deceiving myself for so long. I was also overjoyed because I had broken the cycle of self-deception. I had a new understanding that would allow me

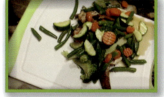
I chopped up a single bowl of vegetables and chicken

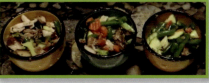
I filled three small bowls, started eating this way and lost 10 pounds in 10 days

to be successful at taking care of myself at a super high level.

The first step toward taking control of your health is to stop lying to yourself. When Doug told me I needed to control my portion sizes, he was really saying to me, "Paul, you're lying to yourself about what you're eating. Stop deceiving yourself." His words set me up for my current success. If you're not giving yourself truthful information, you're not going to get the results you want. Stop lying to yourself. Stop deceiving yourself. Your self-deception is holding you back.

The One Thing:
Self-deception holds you back

2secondlean.com/lh-11

Chapter 12

The Picture Diet

When I learned about Lean and the idea of continuous improvement, I immediately embraced its simplicity. The goal of Lean is to improve operational efficiency by eliminating 8 wastes (overproduction, transportation, inventory, defects, over-processing, motion, waiting and waste of employee potential). Lean compels you to make improvements by making things more simple.

Part of why I like Lean so much is that Lean solutions to problems are often elegant. Elegance appears when things come together in a process without a lot of struggle involved. Lean solutions are simple, visual, easy to execute and most people understand the concepts immediately when you show them. That is my idea of elegance.

Throughout my Lean Health journey, I needed an elegant solution for how I monitor and share what I was eating with others. People I met would always ask me how I was getting these incredible health results. When I told them it was easy, they asked if I would help them. I promised them that every time I ate, I would take a picture of the food and send it to them, if they would reciprocate. That way, they could see what good food looks like and we could hold each other accountable to eating healthier. I dubbed this new technique, "The Picture Diet."

The Picture Diet is an elegant solution because it allows you to monitor what you eat without needing to write everything down. All you have to do is pull out your smartphone and take a picture of the food you're eating. Voila! You have a record you can reference so that you know the quantity and quality of the food you are eating.

Every day, I do The Picture Diet with people all over the world. They send me pictures of the food they're eating, because it's fun and it shows all the different kinds of healthy foods that are available. I have a plethora of pictures of all these fantastic foods that are completely healthy. *(Go to the link at the end of this chapter to watch The Picture Diet videos)*

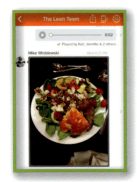

I use The Picture Diet wherever I go. If you opened up the picture gallery on my iPhone, you would see hundreds of pictures of all the different foods that I eat and I think, "Wow! Look how healthy Paul is eating." When I'm traveling in Southeast Asia, the variety of different fruits that are available are staggering. I love to taste and eat every one of them, and every time I do I think to myself how lucky I am that I have fallen in love with all these beautiful plant-based foods and get to enjoy all their tastes and smells. One of my favorites is the durian, a smelly fruit that is popular in Thailand. A durian is about the size of a small watermelon. It has big thorns all over it, and inside are many custard pods that you pull out and eat. Once you get past the initial odor, the creamy, custardy texture inside makes it one of the most wonderful foods ever. I'm always snapping a picture which reminds myself and others that eating fruits and vegetables as your primary food will do wonders for your health.

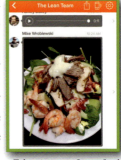

We all need an accountability model. We need a reinforcement system for guiding our behavior.

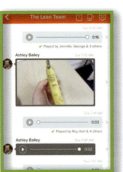

The Picture Diet is as easy as holding your phone above the plate of food you're about to eat, taking a picture and texting it to a group of people, so everyone is accountable. There are no logs to keep. It's just simple and fun. Just like Lean.

Take pictures of your food and send them to each other

Some of you may want to add another layer of accountability to The Picture Diet. For example, I have a very good idea of how many calories I take in every day, but I still feel tempted to lie to myself sometimes about how much

-60-

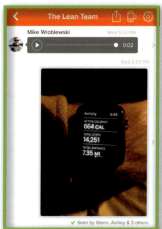

I am eating. Rather than take the chance of compromising my health, I use the MyFitnessPal App to log everything I eat. This adds a little bit of complexity, but not much.

So, keep it simple. Find a friend who wants to do The Picture Diet with you, then start snapping pictures and sharing them. You're going to be shocked at how effective it is.

> ## THE ONE THING:
> ### A PICTURE IS WORTH
> ### A THOUSAND WORDS

2secondlean.com/lh-12

Chapter 13

Lean PD App

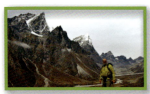
1 day before the 100 year blizzard

Doug, my trainer

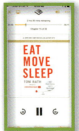
The book that started it all.

Before we go any further, here is a quick recap of what has happened in my life over the last year. I went to Everest Base Camp in October and learned about the book "Eat Move Sleep" by Tom Rath. After reading Rath's book, I began approaching my health differently and started to see positive results.

Shortly thereafter, I started exercising with Doug Scoggins, my trainer who taught me four things:
1. I didn't know how to workout;
2. I can bury a ton of vegetables in a smoothie;
3. I can age in reverse if I take care of myself; and
4. There are no excuses for not taking care of my body.

Doug is a high-powered executive with a large company, yet he finds time not only to work out himself, but to train other people and busy executives throughout our community. Needless to say, Doug taught me a lot. In January, I went surfing and did fantastic because of Doug's training. *(Go to the link at the end of this chapter to watch my surfing videos)*

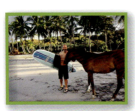
Surfing in Costa Rica

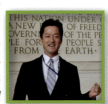
Mr. Harada

Then, in March, I boarded a plane to go to Japan with Norman Bodek, who taught me the Harada Method, a methodology for establishing good habits that was developed by Takashi Harada. In Japan, we met Mr. Harada and had an all-day training session with him that was fantastic. The biggest lesson from the training session was that the habits you do on a daily basis determine the outcomes in your life.

One of my all-time favorite concepts is that "the great equalizer in life is time." Every human being gets the same 24 hours in the course of a day. What we do with those 24 hours determines who we are and how effective our lives will be. Wouldn't it be nice if there was a way to be more thoughtful, more deliberate and deliver more value during that time? The Harada Method is an effective system, but is a bit too complicated for me, so I took some of Harada's ideas and simplified them down to a process I call Lean PD, which is short for Lean Personal Development. *(Go to the link at the end of this chapter to watch my Lean PD video)*

Lean PD
A simple and elegant way to develop powerful daily habits

The Lean PD App (available in the App Store and Google Play) asks you to create a list of tasks you want to perform every day within a group of categories such as health, spirituality, exercise and leadership, among others. If you have 50 habits you want to practice, you list them and check them off as completed so you can easily see the things you have done each day.

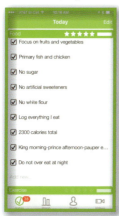

My food check list

Here's an example. One of the categories on my list is Food, and one of the habits in that category is, "No white flour, no sugar, no soda, all fruits and vegetables, primary protein is fish, with chicken as secondary." I don't check off every one of my habits each day, however, I have not missed this one yet. Knowing I would have to admit to cheating on my eating goals has kept me on task, even if I'm the only one who would know about the transgression.

Beyond daily habits, Lean PD also encourages you to set what Jim Collins, in his book "Good to Great," calls a "big hairy audacious goal." It is a good idea to really stretch yourself to pursue a long-term goal, even if it seems out of reach. My goal is to make the world a better place by teaching Lean concepts to an entire country. I want to work with the leader of a nation to bring Lean and all the elements of Lean problem solving to the entire country, in order to show what could happen to

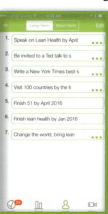

My long-term goals

the world if we worked in a thoughtful way toward solving our problems.

In a previous chapter, I talked about the idea of elegance. One of the things that I wanted very much to build into the Lean PD App was the idea of elegance and simplicity. The App automatically logs tasks as incomplete, all you need to do is check the ones you completed and every night at midnight, the whole thing resets, so you start fresh every day. It is very elegant and simple, with very little management required. The Lean PD App allows you to view your daily, weekly, monthly and yearly progress so you get the big 40,000-foot-view. It graphically shows you how you're performing in every category, so you know exactly where you need to improve.

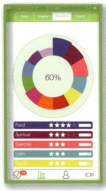

My progress graph

Much of this book is dedicated to the idea of deliberate practices. If you want life to be great for you, you have to be deliberate about the way you approach it. The Lean PD App helps you be very deliberate about the things you eat and about the habits you're developing on a daily basis. By implementing these new habits in my life, I've improved more rapidly and effectively than ever before. In addition to improving my health, these habits have developed my intellect and leadership, too. If you're pre-disposed to wanting to check things off and develop some healthy habits, the Lean PD App might be a great tool for you. It is simple, elegant and effective...everything we strive for when implementing Lean.

THE ONE THING:
CREATE A GREAT PROCESS AND FOLLOW IT

2secondlean.com/lh-13

Chapter 14

To Log or Not to Log?

Keeping track of everything you eat is a critical component of Lean Health. Most people don't want to do it because they think it is difficult, tedious, or just a waste of time. However, if you are serious about wanting to lose weight, you greatly increase your chances of success by writing down everything you eat. When I started on my health journey, I did not know if logging all my meals helped that much, but I've learned that if I record things, it is much harder to lie to myself. I have a 54-year history of distorting the facts when it comes to my diet. In the past, I could say I wasn't eating too much, but I had no way to know for sure. Once I started recording everything, I knew exactly whether I was sticking to my calorie intake goals or not.

One of the tools I use to log my meals is the MyFitnessPal App, a diet tracking and calorie counting App. The MyFitnessPal App lets you input exactly what you eat at every meal and keeps track of calories, carbohydrates, proteins, fats and other nutritional information over time. It also keeps your health data such as weight and exercise if you want it to. *(Go to the link at the end of this chapter to watch my MyFitnessPal video)* I started to use the App in 2013, though at first, I didn't get the results I hoped for. When I looked at a graph of my weight over time, I was shocked to see that between 2013 and October 2014 (when I went to Phuket), I had not lost much weight. The graph was basically flat.

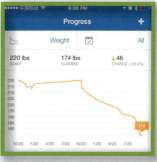
When I started logging "accurately" I started losing weight.

After going to Phuket and reading Tom Rath's book, I started to log my meals more regularly, but not as much as I should have. The tipping point came when my friend Doug told me I needed to control my portion sizes. After that, I became much more consistent in recording my meals and found it easier to lose weight. I finally admitted I was not being honest with myself when I logged my meals, and the MyFitnessPal App was the tool that helped me do that.

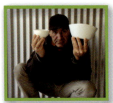
Portion size

The MyFitnessPal App works because it helps you create something called standardized work, another Lean concept. In Lean Manufacturing, we set up processes so that we do them the same way, every time. When we make a particular product, we follow each step in the exact sequence they were set up. The processes have been scrutinized and refined to deliver quality and consistency each and every time.

In Lean Health, I created a standardized process where I eat 2,400 calories a day, every day. I have very little variation, and the consistency has dramatically helped me. That's why I weigh 169 pounds today instead of 220 pounds.

The MyFitnessPal App is not the answer to all your weight problems. Recording your food intake alone does not guarantee you will lose weight. You can record everything you eat, but if you're eating the bad stuff, you're not going to lose weight. The key is being able to consistently record the great food you're eating. Nevertheless, the MyFitnessPal App is very helpful, and I have a couple of recommendations about how to get the most out of it.

First, do not allow the App to link the number of steps you take with your calorie intake. Every day, you want to get 10,000 steps, which you can monitor with some type of pedometer or fitness tracking device (I use a FitBit). If you let it, the MyFitnessPal App will take the information from your device and adjust your daily calorie limit. This includes automatically increasing the number of calories you can eat if you exercise more. For example, if I am allotted 2,400 calories for the day but I walk 20,000 steps, the App will tell me I can eat an extra 1,500 calories that day. When I first started using the MyFitnessPal App, I would take this guidance and

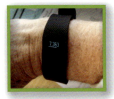
My FitBit that I wear everyday

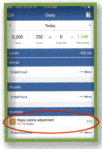
Notice how it added in 373 calories for my 10,000 steps. I always delete these.

go eat 1,500 more calories. You might be able to guess what happened. I didn't lose much weight. This is why I don't sync the MyFitnessPal App with my FitBit, because I do not want to be told I can eat more calories.

The second helpful technique is to always log calories on the high side. I used to be really good at avoiding this. I would find a chicken stir-fry meal that said it had 300 calories when I knew darn well it was probably 450 or 500 calories. I used to record the lower number, but now I do just the opposite. If I see something has 350 calories but I think it might really have 400 or 500, I'll log the higher number because I want to remove any possibility of eating too much.

Ninety-five percent of the people who have tried to mimic what I'm doing are unwilling to log their food. I believe this is because they are intimated by the process or they don't want to be bothered. Avoid this mind-set! Do not be afraid to be honest with yourself. People who log their food in conjunction with the other steps I've talked about in this book are wildly successful. You will be too.

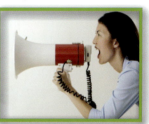

For the love of God, Log your food! It's not hard! It only takes a second.

THE ONE THING:
LOG IT & LOSE IT

2secondlean.com/lh-14

Chapter 15

Racing in the Rain

In earlier chapters, I said that if there was one word to describe Lean Health, it would be Ferrari. The Ferrari is an international symbol for quality, but I have to admit, I'm a Porsche guy. I have a special affinity for Porsche because the Toyota Production System (a.k.a. Lean) was utilized in the year 2000 to turn the company around. By using Lean in their manufacturing process, Porsche improved so much it became one of the best car manufacturers in the world.

Another reason I like Porsches so much is I have spent many hours learning how to *really* drive them. About 5 years ago, a German friend of mine who is really into racing Porsches invited me to attend the Porsche Sport Driving School with him in Birmingham, Alabama. At that time, I had no interest in racing cars. I wasn't a car guy, I was a plane guy, a pilot who got his kicks at 27,000 feet and 300 mph. But I thought, what the heck, I might as well learn something new. So I traveled to Birmingham for a three-day course to learn how to race high-performance cars. *(Go to the link at the end of this chapter to watch Porsche racing video)*

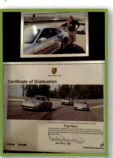
Learning how to race in the rain

Porsche Sport Driving School is not just a bunch of middle-aged men going out there and running cars into the ground without a clue of what they're doing. They educate you on the capabilities of each model of Porsche, and provide intensive training on how to drive them. The express goal is teaching you how to fully enjoy their high performance machines...and there is a lot to enjoy.

If you have never sat behind the wheel of a true high-performance car, the power, the control, and the handling are hard to believe. After a few minutes behind the wheel, I went from being a guy that didn't think much about cars to someone who loves driving high-

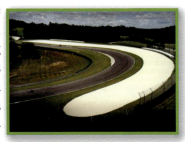
Barber Motor Speedway

performance cars. The whole time I was racing on the track, I was thinking to myself, "How do these engineers pull this off?" I never believed you could drive a car over a hundred miles an hour, take it into corners and have it stick to the road like glue. I did not understand how you could rev the engine to over 6,000 rpms and the car would just keep hammering down.

I remember one of the instructors telling me, "You don't have to worry about hurting these things. They are designed to be driven to the limit. They are so well-engineered that all we do is change the oil and put tires on them." I thought to myself he must have been wrong and that we were abusing those cars by riding them so hard. "Not to worry," he said, "they're designed to do this."

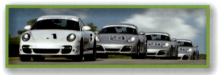

Lining up at Porsche Driving School

All the instructors were professional race car drivers from around the world who came to Birmingham to teach at the school. My particular instructor was Brazilian and he looked like Fabio. He was a good-looking guy, about 6'4", and wow, did he know how to drive. He told us when he left Atlanta for Birmingham that morning for the two-hour drive it was raining really hard. He was driving his Porsche 911, traveling well in excess of 80 miles an hour, and was obviously annoyed by how slow the drivers around him were going. "I don't know why people freeze up when it starts to rain," he said. "You can drive just fine. You just need to know how to do it." I thought it was easy for him to say, being a professional race car driver, but I would learn later that afternoon he was right.

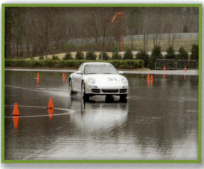

Racing in the rain

One of the many disciplines I learned at Porsche Sport Driving was "racing in the rain," where they flood an entire race course with an inch or two of water before you drive on it. Then the instructors pull out their stopwatches and say, "go race the course." As you can imagine, you can't race the normal way in these conditions. You have to feel the car like you've never felt the car before. You have to understand exactly when the wheels are about to lose contact with the track and know when to ease off the gas or the brake. As you go into the corners, you have to know exactly how much momentum to carry and exactly when to start and stop braking. After a couple of hours, I was getting pretty good at racing in the rain, and I understood why my instructor thought people did not need to slow down so much when it rained. If you know how to drive in those conditions, you can manage very well.

My training paid off in ways I never could have imagined. About six months after returning from my third trip to the driving school (yes, I became a little addicted to it, even though I wasn't a car guy), I was driving down the road at eight o'clock in the morning with my son and another colleague in my Lexus LX470, a big SUV. It was winter, and there was black ice on the freeway, though I did not see it. I had just left Bellingham and was going about 70 miles an hour when I came around a corner where there was quite a bit of shade. As I rounded the corner, a fourteen-car pileup, including a big fire engine, blocked the road in front of me.

I tapped the brakes and my car went into a full 360-degree spin. The car in the fast lane next to me did the same thing. It was not a pretty picture, two cars, moving at 70 miles an hour down the road, spinning side by side, approaching a fourteen-car pileup.

It seemed like somebody was going to get killed, but then all my training kicked in. I didn't even have to think about what I was doing. I tapped my brakes again and I put in a small steering correction, which stopped my spinning for a split second, just enough to get by two cars crashed into each other in the middle of the road.

I was not out of the woods yet. The car next to me collided with a car in the middle of the road, and I was headed right for several cars that were crashed into each other. A quick tap-tap on the brakes to reposition my car allowed us to miss another three car pileup and the fire truck. A third tap of the brakes and we missed another car. Then another one. Finally, one last tap put us gently into the divider where we came to a rest without hitting anyone. It all happened in a blink of an eye and my friend Marc Urban, sitting next to me, looked over and said, "How in the hell did you do that?" The answer is, I was fully attuned to the performance characteristics of the vehicle I was driving, and I understood how to operate it at a high level.

Having good technology helped too, which reminds me of a good health lesson. When you have a car like a Porsche or a Lexus that is beautifully engineered and designed for high-performance, you can really do some amazing things. A year after starting my new health regime, that's the way I look at my body. I don't carry much fat at all. Before, when I carried a lot of weight, everything was just a big mosh pit. I would put stuff into my mouth and not know what was happening to my body. Now, I'm pretty much stripped down to a lean machine and I feel everything I put into my body. Every piece of food that goes into it, I literally feel and register the results of it. When I reflect on this now, I think how I wasted so many years with dulled senses.

Having a body that carries a lot of excess fat is like having a Porsche and then strapping on saddle bags all over it, mounting a roof rack on top and bashing in the front fenders so the aerodynamics are gone, and then saying, "Hey, this is a wonderful sports car." A performance car is not intended to run like that, but that's exactly the way most of us run and manage our bodies.

Do you think I'm wrong? Start observing people's shopping habits the next time you are in a grocery store. Observe what is in their carts. I see piles and piles of processed foods. In contrast, my cart is now full of fresh fruits, vegetables, fish and chicken. The checkers frequently seem surprised by how healthy I eat.

Today, I feel like I'm so in tune with my health. It's almost hard to comprehend how integral my health is to my psychology and everything about me. I enjoy my health completely. I enjoy my body completely. No different than when I look at my Porsche, I say, "Wow! What a machine."

This is the path to an unhealthy life ... the pit stop for Pintos

Our bodies are intended for a lot more performance than most of us have ever understood. I spent a lot of years in a dulled-down, high-performance machine only going 30 mph when I could have been pulling 2 G's at 100 mph. I did not respect the high-performance racing machine I had been given.

Recently, I was talking to a friend of mine, Ty Lane, about Lean Health and about his own journey. Ty is doing the same things that I am, and he was a little frustrated because he had plateaued and really hadn't lost the weight he wanted. I said, "Ty, once you figure it out, it's going to be really simple. Just walk into the grocery store and look around. Everything you see is packaged. There is one section for the fruits and vegetables and a portion of the meat department with the fish and the chicken. That is the good stuff. The rest of it is all there to undermine you. If you can strip away all the other stuff and focus on where the health value is added, you're going to understand your high-performance vehicle like you've never understood it before."

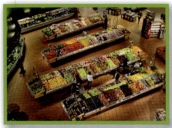
This is the path to exceptional health . . . the pit stop for Ferraris

Just like a Porsche (or a Ferrari), your body was made for high performance from day one. Few people who buy Porsches modify them because they are ready when they come out of the factory. They just need the proper fuel, oil and tires to keep them running. Similarly, your body only needs the right food, exercise and rest to keep it in shape. Stop tinkering with it by adding a bunch of accessories, processed food and other junk to it. Start treating it like it's a purebred, give it what it needs, and you too will be ready to race in the rain.

THE ONE THING:
YOU DON'T KNOW YOUR BODY, AND WHEN YOU DO, YOU WILL BE SHOCKED AT THE HIGH PERFORMANCE MACHINE YOU HAVE BEEN GIVEN

2secondlean.com/lh-15

Chapter 16
The Voice of Others

In the Lean world, we always talk about "Genchi Genbutsu" or "go and see." This phrase means that a manager should go to the shop floor to observe and talk to the people working on the line, in order to understand the processes taking place there. The workers are the ones who have to "do the work," and are thus the best source of information for how the process works.

So far, this book has talked a lot about my own Lean Health journey, but there are many others who have watched what I've done and are following a similar path. In this chapter, we hear about them and their valuable perspective. One of them is Dana May, a very close friend of mine. Dana was with me when we flew out of Everest Base Camp that eventful day in October 2014. He is 65-years-old, and if you look at him today, you would say he's in pretty good shape. When we were on Mount Everest, though, he weighed about 245 pounds, overweight for his 6'5" frame. He also has type-2 diabetes, the consequences of which are potentially very severe (blindness, limb amputation, erectile dysfunction, dementia and a number of other serious consequences). Like me, he had tried many different approaches to better health and every one of them ended with no long-term sustainable habits and definitely not great health.

Over the course of several months, Dana watched my transformation but resisted my prodding to follow the same health regimen. When we traveled to Costa Rica for surf camp, he saw how I chose to not smoke cigars with him, because for the first time, I was not interested in doing anything to compromise my health. Dana also saw how my training with Doug Scoggins had prepared me for success on the surfboard, yet he was still not ready to commit to doing what I was doing.

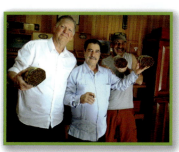

Three months into my Lean Health journey, Dana and I at the cigar factory in Costa Rica This was the first time I asked myself, "Do I really want to smoke these?"

It wasn't until we returned to Thailand in June 2015 that Dana finally gave in (I think he got so tired of people saying I looked good as I strutted around the beach with my shirt off, that he finally said, "Damn, I'm going to do what Paul is doing"). While we were there, Dana decided to change his ways and to follow exactly what I was doing, including eating a plant based diet, with 80% fruits and vegetables and 20% fish and chicken.

In a short time, Dana started to lose weight and feel a lot better. Today, he is doing fantastic. His weight is in at 212 and continues to drop. He has the resolve to continue being healthy, whereas in the past, he'd failed many times at many different diets. Today, we might enjoy a glass of red wine as we sit around and contemplate life, but neither of us are even remotely interested in a cigar. Great health is too addicting and too satisfying. Bad food is no longer tempting. I just got off the phone with Dana, after going to a party over the weekend he said to me "I can't believe the garbage that people are putting into their bodies, they are ruining their health." When I ask Dana if he is tempted, "Are you kidding? As far as I am concerned they are eating rat poison. When I get up in the morning I have no temptation to put rat poison in my coffee."

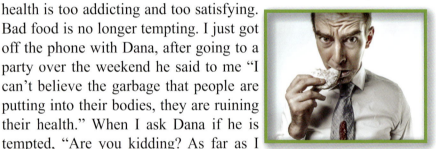

Once you see bad food for what it is, it will never be attractive to you again.

What an amazing transition from a guy who didn't give much thought about what he was eating and putting in his body a year ago, to having total clarity on what is quality food and what is bad food.

Why is the temptation gone? The answer is simple: you learn to see waste in your life. Just like I talked about in my first book, "2 Second Lean," as soon as you begin to see all the waste you produce every day, you're inspired to eliminate it and improve the quality of your life. With Lean Health, once you see all the foods that are destroying people's health, you are compelled to eliminate it. When you go to a party and you see people drinking themselves under the table and gorging themselves on desserts, or you see their guts hanging over their belts, you think, "Of course, look at what they're eating! It's nothing but waste." Once you see bad food for what it is—waste—it cannot be unseen!

Eliminating waste works. By changing his habits, Dana has his diabetes completely under control with no medication and he has significantly reduced his risk of the aforementioned problems. He has a new lease on life, all because of a very simple Lean process applied to health. He is emphatic that he feels like he had to give up nothing and that his new health journey has done nothing but give back to him.

It doesn't matter where you are with your health, you can always get better. Alex and Paloma, who I introduced in Chapter 1, have also made great strides. When I sat with them on the evening I decided to write this book, anyone would have looked at them and said they were the picture of health. Still, they saw the benefits of trying a new way of thinking about food and taking care of their bodies. Since then, Alex has lost 14 pounds and Paloma has lost 8 pounds. They are feeling the best they've ever felt, just by making a few simple changes. Paloma's mother even started the program. She lost 4 pounds and has noticed a sharp reduction in the number of migraines she suffers!

I was chatting with Alex about his results, and he told me something very compelling. "In your book, '2 Second Lean,' you wrote that money suffocates creativity. Conversely, if you do not have a lot of money, you must come up with creative solutions to problems," he said. "The constraints of the Lean Health environment stimulate my creativity. For example, when I walk into a roadside stop where it looks like there aren't any options for healthy eating, I could just give in and buy some junk food. However, because I want to maintain my Lean Health regimen, I find myself being very creative. I ask the clerks behind the counter if they have some fruit or vegetables anywhere, and invariably, they are willing to help me."

Alex said, "Some viable solution almost always comes up. At one roadside stop, the only thing that was available was lasagna. It had a lot of nice tomato sauce and some meat sauce, so I ordered it and ate all the filling between the layers of pasta. My colleagues looked at me like I was crazy, but then they realized what I was doing. 'Look at you!' They said. 'You've lost so much weight, you look great!' I looked at them and said, "Yeah, I know. I'm totally committed."

Filipe is one more recent convert to Lean Health principles. At 35-years-old, his trim stature made him look like he was in perfect health, although in reality he had low energy levels and poor physical shape. Compared to how he feels today, he looks back and realizes he was living like a thin zombie!

Six months ago, Filipe and his father, Tino, came to my company from their native Portugal to visit us for a week of Lean learning. In that time, Filipe got to see my eating habits close up. We made green smoothies, voluminous amounts of fruits and vegetables, and he watched my exercise routine. Most importantly, Filipe saw how serious I took my health and the health of others around me. It's worth noting that we have guests from around the world visit FastCap, and instead of serving the cakes and cookies that most companies provide during coffee breaks, we only serve healthy fruits and nuts, with coffee, tea, or soda water to drink. At lunchtime, we take our guests to Chipotle for fresh, high-quality food and if they follow my lead, a salad.

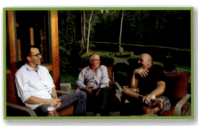

Filipe, his father Tino, and I on there visit to the US in 2015

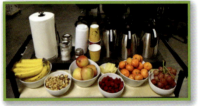

Our guests get served the healthiest food

Filipe returned to Portugal with a new purpose. Six months later, he is running 20 minutes a day and eating fruits, vegetables and healthy smoothies every morning. His cholesterol, which has never been below 205 mg/dl, is now 168. Feeling better than ever, Filipe has more energy and is loving the idea of making small improvements every day to enhance both his company and his health.

Another success story comes from the Lean Summit 2015. I invited 45 of my Lean leadership friends from around the world, and for 3 days we collaborated at my home, at my business and on a hike up Winchester Mountain (elev. 6,521 ft.). One of the people in the group was George Trachilis. George is a fellow Greek and a big guy himself, weighing in at 308 pounds (he's 5'10"). George pushed himself to make it up the

Day 1 Summit At our home

mountain with us, but it wasn't easy. As he pointed out, everyone else had one body to move up the mountain, but he had the equivalent of two bodies to move.

George saw the results I was having and said he wanted to make some changes in his life. I told him he could easily lose 30 pounds by October. We messaged back-and-forth 3-4 times a day, sharing pictures of foods we were eating. George ate lots of vegetables, fish and fresh food. He did not struggle with the quality of the food as much as the quantity, and as soon as he got that under control, he rapidly lost weight.

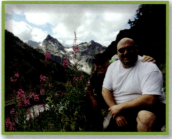

Day 3 Summit
George and I hiking up Winchester Mountain

Two months later, George is down to 265 pounds, he's doing great and he's got complete resolve to bring his weight down to 200 pounds. Just the other day he said, "Paul, this gives me a daily purpose, to continuously improve my health." George even managed to fit into a suit that had not fit for 5 years. Like I said, Lean Health is **aging in reverse**—even our suits are a testament to that!

Once you start down the road toward Lean Health, you gain a sense of clarity about how to best improve your body. You eat healthy, respect your body and cherish your health. Other approaches allow the occasional soda or piece of cake, but this is dangerous. There is no middle ground. The clarity of the Lean Health approach makes the difference because it gives you a clear disdain for those things that undermine your health.

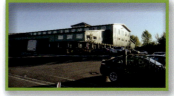

Day 2 Summit
FastCap

Furthermore, the perception that unhealthy foods are enjoyable is really questionable. They bring no lasting satisfaction and you eventually feel miserable after you've eaten them. Contrast that to eating a delicious apple or fresh grapes or crispy carrot

Day 3 Summit
The leadership team at Winchester Mountain

sticks. Quality food is a quality experience from start to finish. There are no negative side effects and only a huge upside. As you learn to appreciate these foods, they will actually be much more enjoyable and satisfying than any piece of German chocolate cake or bowl of Italian ice cream.

You want to be great, not just good. When was the last time you went to a concert because there was a "good" musician playing or a sporting event because you wanted to see a "good" player? We go and watch because we all love what is great, what is remarkable. I have fallen in love with remarkable health and you can too!

As I said in the opening chapter, there are no smoke and mirrors here, there are no diet pills, no books to buy. I will post all this information online along with my videos for free for anyone who wants it. You do not need to buy any special food. All you need is a heavy dose of common sense about how to take care of yourself and then you can get moving on your own Lean Health journey.

THE ONE THING:
BE ALL IN

2secondlean.com/lh-16

Chapter 17

Roadblocks

As I finished up this book, I was talking with a few of my friends. Glen in Pennsylvania, George in Canada, and Ty down in Texas. We were chatting about the difficulties everyone was having while trying to change their health patterns and adopt a Lean Health lifestyle. One challenge for everyone was the tendency to eat in the evenings after dinner.

"I'm struggling with roadblocks," said Glen. "In the evening, I walk into the kitchen and I start grazing."

"I go into the kitchen and I eat a handful of nuts," added Ty. "Next thing I know, I've eaten 5 handfuls and have blown my calorie intake for the day."

George had a similar issue. "I bake vegetables and I feel like I have to eat them all," he said.

Every one of us, including me, have had roadblocks on our health journey. They are inevitable, but they do not decide our fate. We have the ability to overcome them. To do so, one helpful concept from Lean Manufacturing is "source management." The idea is when you want to attack a problem, you need to ask why at least five times (a.k.a. "the five whys") to really get to the source of the problem.

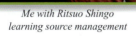

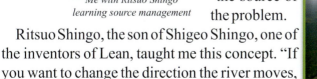
Me with Ritsuo Shingo learning source management

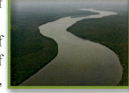
Make the change at the source

Ritsuo Shingo, the son of Shigeo Shingo, one of the inventors of Lean, taught me this concept. "If you want to change the direction the river moves, you must go to the headwaters, the source," he explained. "At the source, you can move a little

It is very difficult to change the direction of a mighty river

soil with your foot and change the entire direction of the river. If you go down to the mouth of the river where it meets the ocean, you must have huge expensive equipment, and it's still going to be very difficult to accomplish." Put simply, the easiest place to fix a problem is at its source.

Let me give you a demonstration of using the five why's to get to the source of the problem:

Once upon a time, Bob's car had an oil plug that leaked and caused an ugly black oil spot on his driveway, making Bob's wife very unhappy! Here are five why questions Bob could ask to get to the root cause of his problem.

Why was the oil plug leaking?
Because the oil gasket material had failed.

Why did the gasket material fail?
Because the purchaser bought cheap gasket material.

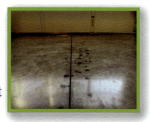

The five whys of leaky oil plug

Why did the purchaser buy cheap material?
Because he was trying to cut costs and save money.

Why was he trying to cut costs and save money?
Because management told him to reduce costs and bring more profit to the company.

Why was management focused on cutting costs and saving money?
Because management didn't understand that building quality is less expensive than cutting costs.

Therefore, the real problem was management and its incorrect focus on cost instead of quality! Management didn't understand the true cost of a defect. Over the long run, focusing on cost at the expense of quality is a shortsighted strategy. When you have to fix a defect, it is like treating someone for a cold in the emergency room—the cost is ten times the cost of doing it right the first time. If you don't believe me, just think about some of the massive recalls that major auto makers have endured the last few years. Wouldn't it have been much cheaper and much simpler to have built the cars without the defects?

This brings us back to my 3 friends. For them, late-night snacking was the roadblock, and we needed to figure out what the true source of the roadblock was. Here is how I would try to get to the source:

Why do we have these nighttime roadblocks?
Because we like to eat.

Why do we like to eat at night?
Because we've developed habits that support nighttime grazing.

Why have we developed these habits?
Because eating makes us feel good, it brings us pleasure and makes us feel satisfied.

Why are we not satisfied?
Our life is not balanced and food may be filling the void.

What is not balanced in our life?
Our health!

Why is our health not balanced?
Because we have developed very strong negative habits that guarantee we will always feel unbalanced and incomplete.

I remember when I was working with a very fit former professional baseball player named Ron. Once, when I was in a colleague's office with him, Ron noticed that the colleague had gained a lot of weight. After the meeting he pulled me aside and said, "Something is going on in his life." I remember that comment because it was very insightful. Ron understood that when we start eating excessively, we are replacing something. We are covering up a hole. We are filling a psychological need with food. We have made food the solution to fill the hole.

In the case of my own roadblock, I was running a medium-size company and was stressed out, so eating felt good. I think that is the root cause of why I would overeat. Something was happening in my head that triggered me to think hey, I need a little pleasure. Let's go into the kitchen and start grazing. This habit became my mindless pleasure.

Managing the source of these roadblocks requires a change in your mental status. If we understand it at this level, I think we have a much better chance of really attacking the issue. This is how I approached the roadblock: First, I understood that for more than 40 years I had developed these bad habits and it would take some time to learn new ones. Second, I knew that I could eat 2,400 calories a day, so I started planning dinner as soon as I woke up. I would think to myself, okay, I'm going to have a nice piece of fish tonight. I'm going to have two or three different vegetables with a sprinkle of parmesan cheese on top and one glass of red wine. After dinner, I'll eat a bowl of blueberries and strawberries, or an apple with cinnamon. Dinner would be 700 calories, a perfectly satisfying way to end the evening. Planning out my evening meal was being mindful instead of being mindless! I didn't let my emotions kick in and run roughshod over all the things I was trying to accomplish. I maintained my determination by looking at myself in the mirror and imagining the next 55-year-old that could be on the cover of Men's Health magazine.

At this point, I would like to make a special appeal to certain people who are reading this chapter. A lot of my friends are CEOs, presidents of organizations who run multimillion/billion-dollar companies and are on a Lean Health journey. We are all smart people. We have built and run organizations that are sophisticated and require a modicum of intelligence to manage. Ladies and gentlemen, don't you think it's time we applied a little intelligence to the way we eat? Don't you think it is time to get the upside benefit of a Lean Health experience?

When I asked myself that question, the only response possible was, "Absolutely. I'm done being stupid." At the same time, I forged an emotional connection with the benefits of being thin and physically fit. I took the emotions causing me to graze at night and rewired them so instead of being connected to the pleasure associated with food, they were tied to the goal of walking in front of that mirror every morning and being happy with the image I see. For 54 years I didn't like what I saw, but those days are over!

      To create the new emotional pathways, we need to use our brains. We've got to stop living emotionally in the way we eat. We've been doing that and it hasn't worked out so well. In addition, we need to preemptively begin to celebrate what it's going to be like walking in front of that mirror and seeing a lean, trim, fit body where the muscle is showing. If we can visualize it in our minds, we can make it happen.

One of my epiphany moments happened about 6 years ago. My wife Leanne had a personal trainer named Valerie. One day, Leanne told me I should have Valerie work-out with me one or two days a week. Sure, I thought, why not. The first thing I told Valerie when I met her was, "I'd love to see my abs."

"Oh, that's really easy," she said. "We've just got to get the fat off of you. The muscles are there," she said, pointing at my abdomen. "The abs are there. They're just covered up by the fat."

It really was that simple.

For each one of you reading this book right now, the abs are there. They're just covered up by fat. We have covered them by grazing and overeating in the evenings (and other times, for that matter). All we need to do is uncover them.

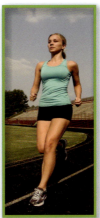

The abs are there. They're just covered up by the fat.

At the end of the day, use your intelligence to overcome your emotions. Set up a plan to get around your roadblocks. Stop eating emotionally. Take those emotions we all have and connect them to something stronger, like seeing the potential that Valerie saw; your abs are there, you just have to uncover them, so someday, when you look in the mirror, you'll be able to say, "Oh baby, look at those abs!"

> ## The One Thing:
> ### Use your brain and get to the root issue

> 2secondlean.com/lh-17

Chapter 18

Lead or Follow

At the end of my first book, "2 Second Lean," I said that Lean is all about leadership excellence. Lean requires leaders at the top who really understand it. Once they do, they will value, respect, teach and train people to collaborate and solve problems. In many regards, I still believe that Lean is about high-level leadership. However, the idea that Lean is all about being a leader comes with a big caveat; we need Lean followers more than we need Lean leaders.

Let me explain. When I was 17, I had the rare privilege of making guitars for two years with Bob Taylor, the founder of Taylor Guitars. This was in the early days of the company, when it was a fledgling startup, far from the celebrated guitar manufacturer it is today. When I started working there, we were making three guitars a day and when I left, the number was closer to 15. Bob was not the world-renowned luthier then that he is today, nor was he swimming in the success he has now. He is an amazing man and I had the privilege of working with him. I paid close attention to everything he did, from tuning a guitar to carving a neck to wiring an electrical outlet. I watched how he thought and how he solved problems. He became my mentor.

For the last 30 years, Bob and I have stayed in contact. He recently told me something that changed the way I view Lean. I was in Kazakhstan and had just finished speaking in front of a group of 1,000 people. I told the audience (as I always do) that Bob Taylor was my mentor. On the way back to the hotel, one of the young men driving me asked who Bob's mentor was. When I emailed Bob to ask this question, his reply gave me something very profound to think about.

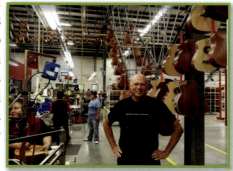

Bob Taylor in his factory

Hi Paul,

I think of a mentor as someone who is a trusted advisor and someone you continually go back to learn from and to problem solve with, someone who has intimate knowledge of something you're trying to learn. I guess I have an old-school mental image of what a mentor is.

Maybe the word has a different meaning nowadays. Maybe we've replaced 'good example' or 'inspirer' or 'most influential' with the word mentor now. Maybe we need a new book called the Two-Minute Mentor! It's a fast world now.

To answer your question, I didn't have a mentor in the way I think of a mentor. I had plenty of two-minute mentors, people who said something to me that were game-changing sentences.

In society, we're always talking about how we need better leaders. I don't agree. We have plenty of good leaders. What we lack is better followers. People don't like to listen these days. Or they don't like to listen and obey.

Bob

We need better followers. His point perfectly captured the key that allowed me to improve my health. All I needed to do was to become a better follower.

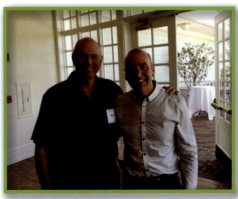
Bob Taylor my mentor

Right now you're probably asking what being a follower has to do with Lean Health. Shouldn't we be leaders in everything we do? Not always. All the information we need to experience amazing health is right in front of our noses. Very wise people have studied it and put it into a form we can understand. The problem is, we are lousy followers. We don't want to listen. We don't want to hear. If we could just stop having what I call "genius disease" (thinking we know everything) and start following some of the great teachers, then we would all have amazing health.

For me, following the prescriptions of Tom Rath and Doug Scoggins made all the difference in the world for my health, and it did not take that long.

As a pilot, I am required to have a physical every year to make sure I meet certain criteria in order to fly my plane. I really, really hated taking the physical. Every year, the doctor would tell me I had high blood pressure. In fact, it was always so high that the doctor would need to turn off the lights and make me lie down to relax. After 15 minutes, he would sneak back in the room hoping that my blood pressure had dropped to the level where he could pass me. Fortunately, I always calmed down enough in those 15 minutes with the lights out and was able to pass my exam and be cleared to fly.

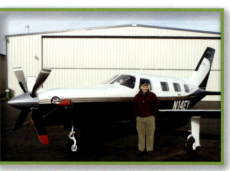

In front of my Jet Prop, I love high performance but I hadn't yet learned the importance of a high performance body.

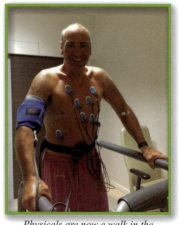

Physicals are now a walk in the park. This was six months into my Lean Health journey.

In the year since my last exam, everything changed. I no longer fear the physical. When the doctor did my annual checkup this year, he told me he has never seen anybody with this type of health at my age. When he asked what I do to maintain my body, I told him how simple it was: 10 minutes of exercise in the morning, a minimum of 10,000 steps during the day and 10 more minutes of exercise in the evening. I eat all fruits and vegetables and fish and chicken and I don't put anything processed into my body—no artificial sweeteners, no sugar, no soda, nothing. He looked at me and said, "Wow, it's so simple, isn't it?"

Yes, it is simple. If you commit to following Lean Health principles, the improvements to health could include: normal blood pressure, blood sugar and cholesterol and the list goes on and on. You won't need to take anything and you will look and feel great. Each one of you reading right now has an opportunity. You can put the book down and forget about it, or you can start now and become a good follower of Lean Health. Head down the path to exceptional health...the choice is yours!

THE ONE THING:
WE NEED GOOD FOLLOWERS

2secondlean.com/lh-18

Chapter 19

Discipline or Intelligence

Frequently throughout my life, people have said to me, "Paul you're so disciplined." Every time they said that, I would think to myself, "Am I really that disciplined? Do I have some special corner on the market on discipline and follow-through?" The more I thought about it, though, I realized it wasn't discipline that I possessed, it was intelligence.

I'm not saying I was super smart, especially when it came to academics. I was always a poor student in school, lucky if I could manage a C in any course. I couldn't take a test to save my life, and I was woefully slow in most open discussions. I was so bad at reading that I read Dick and Jane countless times so that when I read out loud in class, I wouldn't be branded as the class idiot. The only thing I ever excelled at was woodshop.

Still, I was intelligent enough to learn from people with more experience. When I was a young man, I observed my father investing in real estate, even though he didn't have a lot of money. He had a few rental properties that provided a small, but consistent income stream for our family. This additional income allowed us to live comfortably, beyond the salary he made working at General Dynamics.

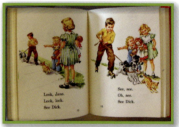
The book I read countless times to avoid embarrassment

Following my father's example, when I graduated from college, I made it my goal to buy one house every year. It would have been easy for my wife and I, both college graduates, to do what our friends were doing; go on nice vacations, buy nice homes and adorn themselves with nice clothes and cars. We did not have a lot of money, but we could have leveraged ourselves and used credit to live a pretty good lifestyle. That's not the path we took. Instead, my wife and I

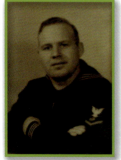
I followed my dad, Harold's example--the value of investing for the future

chose to live frugally in a very rough neighborhood in La Puente, California. I knew if we could live frugally for 10-15 years, the rest of our lives would be much easier. Instead of spending our resources, we invested them. The plan worked. We are very successful financially today. Once again, the question is, were we successful through discipline or intelligence?

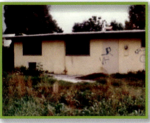

Our humble beginnings in La Puente, CA

My friends would say it was discipline, but I say it was intelligence. I looked at the facts and knew I did not want to struggle when I was in my thirties, forties and fifties, so I made the intelligent decision to invest a good portion of my income into real estate, and it paid off.

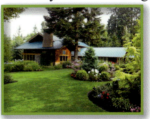

Our current home in Bellingham, WA

Let's fast-forward to the year 2000, a very important year for me and my company, FastCap. At the time, FastCap was doing very well. We had won several business awards, were growing by leaps and bounds, were generating excellent financial results, and were creating so much buzz around town that the president of our bank (which had just granted us a very large line of credit) came to visit for a tour. He was blown away by what he saw and said our business was the best he had ever seen.

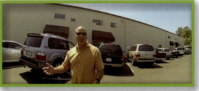

FastCap's first manufacturing plant where we learned about the Toyota production system and Lean manufacturing

Shortly thereafter, I brought in two consultants from Japan to help me manage inventory. They didn't agree with the president's assessment. On the first day, one of them took a look at the factory and told me bluntly, "You're clueless. You don't know what you're doing. You need to learn the Toyota Production System." Intrigued, I hired them to teach us the Toyota Production System. Within a couple months, we completely transformed the entire factory, reducing inventory and drastically shortening our production processes. The amount of waste we eliminated was staggering!

After that, I had to see what Toyota was doing, so I went to Japan and visited the Lexus plant in Kyushu. I could not believe what I saw. FastCap was not just behind Toyota, it wasn't even on the same planet! The trip made me want what Toyota had, a company that functioned at a high level and did not require an enormous amount of management, with happy, fully-engaged, long-term employees. I wanted to stop struggling to run my company and move from being a babysitter to being a leader. When I got back to the U.S., I fully dedicated myself to implementing Toyota Production System (Lean) at FastCap. By doing so, we managed to make a great company even better.

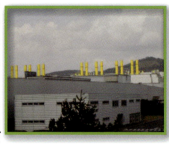

Lexus plant in Kyushu, Japan where I first saw Lean Manufacturing and operational excellence

Today, many people look at me and say, "You had so much discipline to follow through with that, to bring your company to such a high level that everybody wants to emulate what you're doing." I thought, "Was it really discipline?" I am convinced it was not discipline; rather, it was intelligence. I knew what I had, I knew what Toyota had, and I told myself I would not settle in my life until I had what Toyota had. It took some time, but FastCap went from being a good company to a great one and I am now able to focus on being the leader I wanted to be. My intelligence is what got me there.

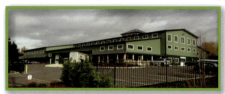

2014 FastCap's new manufacturing plant

Once again, let's fast-forward, this time to 2014, when I learned how to take care of my body, a.k.a. "my customer." For 54 years, I was incredibly ignorant about how to take care of my body. I was, as I said in an earlier chapter, incredibly stupid. I had little understanding about health and was definitely not enlightened about the relationship between my body and my well-being.

That changed when I had an epiphany while reading on the beach in Phuket. I realized that if I put high-quality food into my body in the right proportions, my body would look

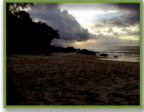

On the beach in Phuket, Thailand

amazing and I would feel fantastic.

When I was attending conferences, I would observe the correlation between what people were eating and how much they weighed. Finally, I put everything together—it was not a coincidence that what people put into their mouths determined how they looked. For the first time, I understood this at an intellectual level, and my intelligence would shape how I acted from then on.

Others have benefited from using their intelligence in this way. My friend Dana is currently on a three week trip to Baja California with 11 of his closest friends from high school. You would think he would be stepping into a lion's den of food and alcohol, and would need a special dose of discipline to stay on his Lean Health journey. I would think the same thing, but we would all be wrong.

Instead of being tempted, Dana told me he is expecting to weigh in four to five pounds lighter when he gets home—after three weeks of partying with his friends! Dana didn't go on this trip with a fortified amount of discipline. He went on this trip with total enlightenment and intelligence, and I know he will maintain his health regimen. Dana called me while he was on his trip and at one point in our conversation, he stepped away from his friends for a minute because he did not want to offend them. He quietly said to me, "Paul, I can't believe the crap these people are putting into themselves. They are destroying their lives! They're destroying themselves with what they're eating and drinking!" Dana's intelligence produces his strength to resist temptation.

If you think you're going to muster up the discipline to carry you to remarkable health, I've got bad news for you...it is not going to happen. If you open up your mind to change and trust your intelligence, everything will change for the future of your health.

The One Thing:
Use your intelligence to succeed

2secondlean.com/lh-19

Chapter 20

Building a Lean Team

When I get ready to speak in front of thousands of people, the first words that often come out of my mouth are, "I have a true confession. I don't like Lean. I love Lean." I say that because Lean delivers so much joy to people's lives. The act of deliberately and continuously improving every aspect of your life—at home, work and play—brings joy to every person I've ever met who understands it and does it.

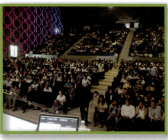

*"I don't like Lean, **I love Lean**"*
Speaking in Kazakhstan

One of the great things about Lean is the sense of community that accompanies the people who do it. Within the Lean community, there are no excuses. There are no victims. There are just people who want to make life better for themselves, their communities, and the world. I have friends around the world who are supportive of me in every regard and would do anything for me, and all of them are involved with Lean. They are all people who love continuous improvement and the joy and collaboration that comes with it.

In Chapter 1 of this book, I told a story about Alex and Paloma, two friends and fellow Lean practitioners. Now I'm going to end the book by talking about them once again.

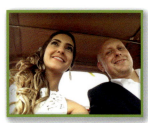

Paloma and Alex

When we were together in Baden-Baden, Germany, visiting Mercedes-Benz, the three of us had a conversation where I revealed that I really wanted to learn how to dance. It was something I had on my bucket list, but I was unsure how to go about it because I was so awkward and clunky. (Side note: One of my favorite television programs of all time is the Seinfeld episode called "Elaine Dancing." It's hilarious. Elaine suffers from the same problem I had. She just cannot move. When she tries to dance, she is very staccato, very angulated and not smooth or rhythmical at all. I laughed so hard at that episode because it reminded me of myself.)

Paloma looked at me, "I'm a Zumba instructor, and I think you should do Zumba."

Having seen the complicated Zumba moves before, I thought to myself, "Wow, that does not sound fun." I looked at Alex, "Do you do Zumba?"

"No," he replied in a stern German accent. Paloma rebuked him. I said, "Come on Alex, you have a beautiful wife. She does Zumba. You've got to learn how to do Zumba."

"Well, I never really gave it much thought," he admitted.

Not wanting to make excuses, I promised I would do it the following day. So, the next morning when I woke up, I opened my MacBook Pro and searched YouTube for beginning Zumba lessons. It was not long before I found a video that showed me the basic moves. Soon, this awkward, clunky man who had never danced before in his life was actually starting to feel the moves.

The next day when Alex and Paloma picked me up, I told them I did Zumba. They did not believe me. "I did," I insisted. "I followed a video on my computer and had so much fun." Both were impressed I had been willing to try it and encouraged me to do it again.

You can understand why continuous improvement is so addictive. When you surround yourself with people who are optimistic, who are steeped in positivity and want to help and encourage one another, it is unbelievable what can happen.

So much has changed in my life over the last year. I love my health. I love my body. I even feel totally comfortable dancing. I would not have said any of that before. I'm appreciative and grateful that I finally figured out how to take care of my health at a high level. I'm appreciative that this new me inspires other people to reach for excellence and to break the mold of mediocrity.

No one is successful on their own, and we need others alongside us. My life is richer because I'm surrounded by an amazing team of Lean people who understand the power of continuous improvement. If you have a group of friends and colleagues dedicated to the idea of improvement, it will push you to continually better yourself. I encourage you to build a Lean team, embrace the idea of Lean Health and get going on one of the most powerful journeys you will ever take.

Speaking of journeys, I was on a recent study mission in Japan, when the leader of our group, Norman Bodek, asked us a question. "What is Japan all about?" He said. Not one of us could answer the question correctly. Finally, Norman revealed the answer with one word: Quality. He told us that the Japanese learned quality from W. Edwards Deming (a famous American researcher, engineer, author and consultant) and on the strength of this quality,

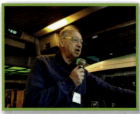

Norman Bodek
"The mind is a wonderful slave, but a terrible master."

Japan became a manufacturing powerhouse. Many of the best brands in the world: Sony, Panasonic, Canon, Nikon, Toyota, Honda, Mitsubishi, Komatsu, Kubota, are all Japanese companies famous for their quality.

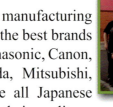

Japan Study Mission 2015
Deepening our understanding of Lean Manufacturing

Quality speaks volumes. At the end of the day, the goal of Lean Health is to build quality into your life. The system helps you fall in love with high-quality foods and reject low-quality foods. Combined with exercise, it will consistently bring you exceptional health throughout your entire life.

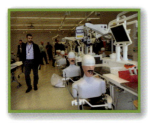

Visiting a Lean dental equipment manufacturer in Japan

To wrap things up, here is one of my favorite stories of all time. A good friend of mine from Germany has a manufacturing company in the United States, and about 15 years ago, he wanted to visit China to see the capacity of factories there and to gauge whether some of his products could be manufactured or sourced there. This was during what people refer to as the "Wild West" days of China. Today, China is one of most technologically advanced and sophisticated places you'll ever go, but 15 years ago, it was pretty crazy. Figuratively speaking, it was like the early days of the American West. A spirit of opportunity filled the air, but the rules were fluid and always changing, so trying to do business there was survival of the fittest.

If you wanted to be successful, you needed help from someone inside China, so my friend set up the two-week trip through a Chinese liaison. When he arrived at the airport, his Chinese guide picked him up in what my friend describes as a "stolen 300 SEL Mercedes." The guide could not speak English, so for 2 weeks, they communicated only with gestures as they drove all over China to visit different manufacturing plants.

While they were traveling, the two ate together frequently, visiting many types of restaurants. The entire trip, this small Chinese guy (about 100 pounds dripping wet) kept taunting my large German friend (6'2" and 210 pounds), goading him to eat some exotic food that the Chinese people love. Each time, my friend resisted. Toward the end of the trip, the two ended up in Beijing. They walked into a restaurant for dinner and the guide motioned toward some silkworms in one of the aquariums nearby. Restaurant entrances often have

Choosing what to eat in a typical Chinese restaurant

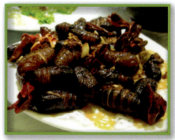

Eating silkworms in China

aquariums full of fish or other small animals from which you choose the specimen you want for dinner that night. He said to my friend, "We get this." My friend was very hesitant but thought, "Man, I just can't be rude the entire trip," so he reluctantly agreed to try them. After ordering the silkworms they went back to their private dining room. When the food came, my friend picked up his chopsticks, grabbed one of the silkworms and popped it into his mouth, swallowing hard to get it down (later, he would tell me it was the most disgusting thing he's ever tasted in his life). Then he looked over at his guide and said, "Okay, your turn now."

His Chinese host looked back at him, and, in perfect English, said, "I don't eat that sh*t!"

That sentence pretty much sums up what this book is about. Are you going to continue to eat the sh*t that has made you fat and sloppy or are you going

It looks tasty, but you might as well go pour sugar and water in the gas tank of your Ferrari

to choose quality and have remarkable health? There really is only one choice. You are the only one in the driver's seat of your Ferrari. You can make the intelligent decision to cut off your old destructive ways and enjoy exceptional health the same way I did. My hope is that you will use what you have learned in this book to experience fantastic life-giving health the rest of your days.

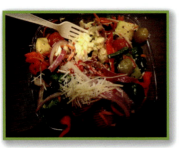

It looks tasty, is tasty and fuels your Ferrari.

The One Thing:
Exceptional Health is all about quality

2secondlean.com/lh-20

A Typical Day for Paul

What exactly does an average day look like for me? I wake up at by at least 5 o'clock, sometimes earlier. Don't be put off by this, it's not because I'm overly disciplined about getting up very early in the morning, it's just that I'm not a big sleeper and I find myself laying in bed at three and four thinking about things, so rather then do it too long I get up and get going. A simple idea is "early money is better than late money." The idea is the earlier you get up, the higher the overall productivity for the day.

I'm very passionate about replying to all my emails promptly and not making anyone wait to get an answer from me. The first thing I'll do before I get out of bed is answer all my emails for 15 or 20 minutes. I use Siri which types all of them very quickly and very efficiently. If the answer requires a more detailed response I always use the audio memo feature and record my voice so the person can hear all the nuances of my reply.

My wife sleeps soundly so she can't hear a thing I do (she just heard me say this and she says, yes I can hear you, I just ignore you). It's 2:37 a.m. when I'm typing this chapter.

Next, I get on my workout clothes and head directly to the coffee machine. I love a hot cup of coffee or tea. Next, I open up the fridge and pull out all the vegetables, then get the blender and begin making my green smoothie. Again, I have a great smoothie video where you can see exactly how I make them. *(Go to the link at the end of this section to watch my smoothie video)* I have 4 stainless steel Contigo 20 ounce containers that I pour the 4 smoothies into. I have a small lunch bag that I take to work so I put 3 of the smoothies in the bag, along with some fruits and any other food that I plan on eating during the day. At this point I'm pretty much ready to start my workout and I'll go to my workout room with coffee and smoothie in hand and sip on those periodically as I'm working out.

I turn up the music really loud. I take my iPhone and tell Siri to shuffle my music. I start with some kind of a mellow song as I begin my stretching and my trunk twists to warm my body up. I'm very reflective during this time thinking about all the great things and about what I'm getting ready to do for my body. I refer to this as being mindful. I read a book "Mindfulness for Dummies" by Shamash Alidina. It is fantastic and I highly recommend it. I'm not going through the motions, I'm fully aware that I'm doing the most important thing I could ever do for my body. I start off by making sure my form is correct, arms flat and level, twisting my core a full 180 degrees. I'm doing this all in front of a mirror. My exercising is for the purpose of allowing my body to operate at the highest level, ensuring a lifetime of high-performance and respect for my Ferrari.

At home I'm able to work out for between 20 and 30 minutes. I really enjoy this time and I always feel amazing at the end of it. I want to emphasize I am rocking and rolling with the music. I produced a really cool video on my exact workout. I think it's best to watch that, it is only about 2 minutes long. *(Go to the link at the end of this section to watch my workout video)* I sped everything up so you can see exactly what I do. There is also a video on my work-out routine when I'm traveling. *(Go to the link at the end of this section to watch my travel workout video)* I don't generally have exercise equipment and I quit relying on the hotels to have adequate gyms. If they do, that's great, but for the most part, I do everything in the hotel room. I have my Bose SoundLink Mini with me and I am rocking and rolling in the hotel room. Nobody's ever stopped me or knocked on my door and told me to turn it down. After my work-out routine I do 2 to 3 dance Zumba songs that really get my heart rate up. I love doing this!

After my workout I continue to drink my coffee and smoothie and it takes me about a half hour to get ready in the morning. I leave for work around 6:00-6:30 a.m. Another cool thing that I've learned from a friend of mine who is a world-class athlete is something called "Shoga", which is stretching in the shower with the hot water running on you. I make sure I touch my toes for an extended period of time to make sure that I'm very well stretched out. I'm not sure how much the hot water helps, but it sure feels good. On the drive to work I'm generally listening to a book on tape or putting myself in the correct state by listening to some of my favorite music.

I'm very fortunate that I have a very high performance car and this car always reminds me of the state that I want for my physical body.

At work, I'm on my feet. I have no office and I'm always walking around working with people and helping people do their jobs more effectively. Because I am a Lean maniac and we have such a deeply embedded culture, I will start my day by 3-S'ing my work area, making one small 2 second improvement. At 7:30 a.m. after a half hour of 3-S'ing and helping others with improvements, we have our morning meeting with the entire company. By 8:30 a.m. everyone is at work, including me. I'm always on my phone, answering emails, but throughout the course of the morning, I'm always sipping on my smoothie and a coffee. Around 10 a.m. it is very common for me to be sitting at the break table eating an apple and orange or some other fruit. I log everything I put in my mouth in the MyFitnessPal App. I log my 4 smoothies as 800 calories and I put that in first thing in the morning, even though I generally drink them throughout the course of the day.

At noon I use my Chipotle App and order a salad and go eat it at the restaurant (no waiting). It is very efficient. I often bring food to work such as stir-fry vegetables with fish or chicken. This way I'm eating tons of vegetables at lunchtime, augmented by the protein of fish or chicken. At the end of the day I have walked between 10,000 and 15,000 steps just by walking around our facility.

We have a fantastic gym at our facility and I run up there throughout the day and do 6 pull-ups. It is very difficult to do, but I love this physical challenge. By 3 p.m. I'm at the break table again eating more fruit. By 5:00 p.m. it is very common for me to be eating leftover salad or some leftover stir-fry. Leanne and I generally head home between 5:00 p.m. and 6:00 p.m. We get home and Leanne makes an amazing meal with lots of vegetables and a piece of fish. It is also very common to have one glass of red wine with my evening meal. After dinner I usually have 2-3 handfuls of blueberries or raspberries to round out the day. I try to get in bed as early as 8 p.m. but generally no later than 10 p.m. Leanne and I watch very little TV. It's rare that it's ever on other than in the morning catching the news as we are getting ready. I always make sure to check my Lean PD App and check off everything I've accomplished that day. If I can hit at least 60% to 70% completion, I feel happy. I'm always working to improve but that's pretty doggone good for the aggressive habits that I've laid out for myself. I put on Audible with the sleep timer for anywhere between a half hour and an hour and listen to an audio book as I fall asleep.

It's all pretty simple and straightforward, but it's a great routine that takes excellent care of my health and my mind and I love every second of it. The best part of what I do is I never have a meal or food intake that I'm regretful of—and I mean never! Everything I put in my body is perfect. My mind has changed fundamentally about the way I manage my health.

It's easy and 100% enjoyable

2secondlean.com/lh-day

21 Stages of Lean Health

As you work your way toward excellent health, these are some of the stages you will go through on your journey:

1. You try the process for two weeks and it starts to make sense.

2. You begin to look at processed foods differently and have a small degree of disdain for them.

3. You start to really enjoy eating fruits and vegetables. You're not sure you can sustain a high level of intake, but you try it and you feel better.

4. You continue to lose weight at the reasonable pace of one to two pounds each week. People begin to make comments about how good you look and start asking you what you are doing.

5. You have a growing and intensified disdain for anything processed: flour, sugar, artificial sweeteners, pastries, sodas, sugary drinks, or anything else that would rob you of excellent health.

6. You begin to fall in love with vegetables, fruit, fish and chicken—everything that is nutritious and nourishes your body and improves your health.

7. You simultaneously learn the importance of exercise and movement and these two components become central to your thinking 24/7.

8. The weight comes off steadily but you begin hitting plateaus. You resolve to understand your body at a deeper level, and for the first time, you realize you're eating too many calories. You recognize the importance of counting calories and controlling portion size. You stop lying to yourself about how much you're eating.

9. Eating smaller portion sizes becomes a habit and you drop pounds that you've never been able to lose.

10. You see yourself in the mirror and you ask, "Who the hell is that?"

11. You step up your exercise program and begin to work much more vigorously, doing sit-ups and push-ups to the point of failure. Your body is becoming more and more toned and you start resembling someone on the front of a health magazine instead of an overweight middle-aged person.

12. Nearly every day, someone asks what you are doing to look so fantastic. You resolve to eat fruits and vegetables as your primary foods with chicken and fish as your protein and never put a bad thing in your body ever again.

13. You view your body with great respect because you realize it is vastly superior...an expensive exotic sports car. You would do nothing to harm it, so you protect and nurture it with the best fuel and maintenance at all times.

14. You walk by fruits and vegetables and you get excited because you know they are going to help you be in exceptional physical condition. You trust they will take care of all your health conditions and rid you of problems you've had for many years, so you eat them to satisfy your hunger instead of eating processed food.

15. You reflect back on all the wasted years when you abused your body and did not treat it with proper respect and you resolve to never let that happen again.

16. You look for every opportunity to exercise. You see an elevator as a death machine that keeps you sedentary and adds to your weight problems, so you always take the stairs instead.

17. You consistently make great choices about everything regarding food and exercise. People around you see your actions and want to mimic what you are doing.

18. Your doctor will probably advise you to stop taking all supplements, pain killers and sleep medications, because if you take care of your body properly with both food and exercise, you will have exceptional health and sleep well.

19. Your mind is completely changed about food and health and you get great satisfaction from finally discovering what excellence in health is all about.

20. You're never hungry anymore. You eat because you know it's time to nourish your body. The hunger pains are gone forever. This is perhaps one of the craziest realities I've ever experienced. I spent my entire life being hungry and satisfying those urges by filling my mouth with junk that made me more hungry. I cannot overemphasize how gratifying it is to fill my stomach appropriately and timely with the correct amount of good-quality food.

21. You start sharing your success with the world. I produced multiple videos on how I lost weight and achieved exceptional health. I am in better physical shape than when I played football in high school. Go to Lean Health YouTube channel to see how I did it.

2secondlean.com/lh-stages

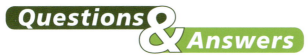

All the answers below are my opinions. I am not a medical professional. This is what has worked for me—no more, no less.

1. How much water should I drink?

Hydration is extremely important—the more the better. I drink four 20 ounce smoothies a day for a total of 80 ounces of liquid. After drinking my smoothies, I shake the container with cold water and drink it so I do not waste any of the nutrients packed on the walls of the thermos. This gives me an additional four cups of water every day and captures a bunch of nutrients I would otherwise be rinsing down the sink.

Additionally, I drink four teas or coffees for another 80 ounces of liquid. Beyond that, I don't measure how much I drink, because I always have a 20 ounce thermos in my hand and am hydrating all day long. Consuming fruit with a high water content (watermelon, oranges, cantaloupe, papayas, grapes, blueberries, raspberries and mangoes) adds to my fluid intake as well.

My trainer, Doug, said that if your urine is a dark color, you are not hydrated enough; it should be light in color. I use this as a rule of thumb and find it to be very accurate.

2. What is your opinion about organic versus non-organic?

The two greatest scams perpetrated on the American public over the last ten years are the front-loading washing machine and paying 2-3 times more for products because they have the word organic on the box. I am not saying that organic is not better, but that is not the issue when it comes to our health.

The real issues are:
- We don't eat enough fruits and vegetables, organic or not.
- We put a bunch of processed crap in our body, organic or not.
- We put way too many drugs and over-the-counter medications in our body that are absolutely not necessary.
- We need to get off our asses and start moving more.
- We need to stop blaming other people for our problems and take responsibility for the things we have control over.

If we took care of these issues, we would solve 95% of the health problems people have. Eating only organic food will not solve your health problems.

3. Should I buy the pro version of the MyFitnessPal App?

It is not necessary, but it can be useful. For three years, I've used the free version and just ignored the additional calorie allotment that shows up when FitBit sends my exercise statistics to the MyFitnessPal App. Nonetheless, I bit the bullet and paid $49 for a year's subscription to see how the paid version works. So far, I'm very happy with the decision. I like that I never have to be distracted by those additional calories. I also like a few other features that come with the pro version. At the end of the day, for me to spend $49 a year to have an enhanced and better experience for maintaining near-perfect health is worth it to me.

4. What if my wife doesn't support what I'm doing?

You cannot use that as an excuse. Once you see bad food and excessive food for what it is, a direct path to poor health and a poor quality of life, it doesn't matter who supports you or not. You will have the resolve to make this work.

5. What should I do if I'm always hungry?

If you're always hungry, you're doing something wrong. You should never have hunger pains, just a gentle nudging that says it's time to eat something. You might be eating foods that are making you hungry—starches, bread, pasta, refined sugar, or artificial sweeteners. You may also have stretched your stomach in the same way that people elongate their earlobes to fit those large oversized hoops in them.

To get your stomach back into shape, you're going to need to stop eating 4 times more than you need to. I recommend using your intelligence and your reasoning to ask yourself if you really need to eat 4,000 or 5,000 calories a day. I'm a big guy with a lot of muscle and I perform at the highest level on 2,400 calories a day. In the past, I would easily eat 5,000 to 6,000 calories a day for no reason other than sheer stupidity.

There are a couple of strategies that can help you manage your hunger in a better way. You should always carry an apple, a piece of fruit, or small bag of nuts with you, so that the moment you get hungry you can eat something healthy. Also, you should always have a thermos full of liquid nearby so you can immediately drink some if you feel hunger pains coming on between mealtimes.

6. How do you exercise when you travel?

Everything for me is so simple and straightforward:
- I make sure I move 10,000 steps a day by watching my FitBit
- I wake up every morning and rock out to Taylor Swift using my Bose SoundLink Mini speakers while I do my 10 minute workout routine

which includes Zumba dancing for 2-3 songs
- 100 trunk twists
- 100 push-ups (or to exhaustion, whichever comes first)
- 200 sit-ups/crunches (or to exhaustion)

7. Are you against modern medicine or modern drugs?

I am the biggest proponent of modern medicine and grateful for our amazing medical system. I am planning on living well beyond 100-years-old because of the advancements in medical technology. Having said that, it does not mean we should use technology to avoid our responsibility to take care of our bodies. We must get the fundamentals right and then leverage technology and medical advancements to support a longer and healthier life.

8. Where does your passion come from?

It probably comes from the fact that I never felt I was gifted. Then I discovered life itself was a gift, and now I see the world as positive and moving forward even though it has many problems. My overall view is that, compared to what people had 100 years ago, we are lucky to live in the most amazing times.

9. Why do you think it took you so long to figure your health out?

The best answer I can give is that I was 'uncomfortably content.' I was uncomfortable with my health, but not enough to take necessary action. I did not apply the standard of excellence to my health like I did everything else in my life. I read many books about health, but none of them made having exceptional health simple and comprehensive. It wasn't until I read Tom Rath's book that I put it all together.

This is the only thoughtful answer I can give to why it took me 54 years! I promise I was trying to figure it out. As I reflect back on the time I spent developing my company, my leadership and my communication skills, I know that if I would have given equal time to learning how to have excellent health, I would have discovered this much sooner. Ironically, excellent health would also have improved those other categories significantly, but I just didn't put it all together.

10. How do you get your smoothies when you travel?

You have to be creative sometimes. When I went to Costa Rica for a month, I had access to a blender, so I was able to maintain my routine. I did take my own blender on a different trip, but finding and handling the ingredients was not worth the trouble, so now I load up on vegetables and fruit during my regular meals. If I have someone at a café or restaurant make me a smoothie, I'm very emphatic they do not add sugar. Many shops and restaurants put sugar and other stuff in the smoothies to make them taste better, but I watch them like a hawk to make sure they don't.

If you have your own car and are on a road trip, it is feasible to make your own smoothies. My good friend Dana, who I talk about a lot in this book, just went on a 3 week trip to Mexico and took his blender and a Yeti Cooler. He said he found all the ingredients easily along the way and was able to maintain his smoothie routine. In addition, a lot of the guys that he was traveling with enjoyed and came to love the smoothies as well.

11. Why do you think Lean Health works so well for you?

I looked at the entire value stream of my health (to use Lean terminology), tore up the whole process, threw out everything bad and only left the good stuff. The key to getting healthy has been to get all the following points correct:
- Maintain a focus on fruits and vegetables
- Eat fish and chicken as your primary protein sources
- Disdain and remove everything processed and packaged from your diet, as well as sugar and artificial sweeteners. The only exceptions I can think of would be nuts, sparkling water and cheese (which I don't eat a lot of anymore, but I do enjoy).
- Move 10,000 steps a day
- Include a short, intense muscle-building workout every day
- Treat your body like it's your customer and treat it with respect because it is the reason you're in business

12. Why do you see your body as a customer?

As a successful businessman and entrepreneur, one of the most important ideas I have ever internalized is the importance of loving my customers. I make things they want and improve the quality of their lives. They do me a great favor and keep coming back over and over to buy my products and improve the quality of my life. Your body is your number one customer of all time! Your body needs the services and goods that you provide. Food, shelter, nourishment, intellectual stimulation and spiritual mindfulness. You give it high-quality inputs and it returns a high-quality life to you—this is the law of compensation.

13. How do I start?

You can start by focusing on the three areas that have the greatest impact. First, increase your intake of fruits and vegetables. Second, eliminate processed food from your diet. Third, be very deliberate about walking 10,000 steps every day. Once you've mastered those three, gradually incorporate other suggestions from the book and you will reach your health goals more quickly than you ever dreamed.

14. What are the 3 biggest benefits to being in excellent health?

This may seem a little crazy, but always feeling like every meal was perfect is the first benefit. I never have regrets anymore after I eat and I never feel bloated. So much mindfulness goes into everything that goes into my mouth that fueling up is a perfect experience every day. Perfect taste, perfect nutrition and perfect portion. I am crazy about the idea of getting it right every time.

The second is the praise I receive from others. Everywhere I go, the first thing people say when they meet me is, "Wow, you look amazing!" When you take someone like me who has always been average and transform them into someone who could model with his shirt off at 55-years-old, it is hard to overstate the boost this has given my self-esteem. I do not know any 50-year-olds that look as good as me. Being in such an exclusive group of people makes you feel pretty special and the confidence it gives you is indescribable.

The third benefit is seeing the impact my example is having on other people. The idea that my mindfulness is helping other people is deeply inspiring.

Two additional benefits (because three are not enough!) are being able to wear fewer clothes (I no longer need them to hide my body), and never getting sick. I cannot totally explain why it works, but my consecutive days of not catching a cold or the flu is hard to comprehend.

15. What is the Lean Health credo?

I am the boss of food, it will never rule me, it will only help me. I love everything about it in its most natural unprocessed form. I disdain things that are processed and packaged. Quality food, in exactly the right amount, gives me amazing health and an amazing life!

16. Can you summarize Lean Health in one word?

Ferrari!

Where it all began, Paul's first book on Lean Manufactoring

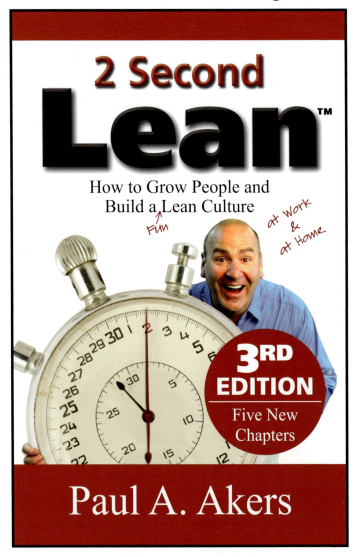

Check out Paul's
2 Second Lean book for FREE
online at 2secondlean.com